DASH Diet Cookbook for Beginners

Delicious Recipes to Lower Blood Pressure

Sophie Nutrify

Table of Content

Introduction

It is getting tough to maintain a healthy lifestyle in the fast-paced life of today's world. Current health diseases have swept millions globally, the most common being high blood pressure or hypertension. The high numbers are rooted in the lack of diet decency, where people cannot regulate what they eat every day due to tight working schedules. Many people find it hard to continue on a diet and eat the exact food every day due to monotony.

In this book, I introduce you to the Dietary Approaches to Stop Hypertension diet — a meal plan developed based on scientific criteria and proven to reduce blood pressure effectively — and tell you more about how to be on this diet. DASH is not just about reducing salt intake; it is balanced nutrition, rich in fruits, vegetables, whole grains, and proteins such as chicken and fish. In addition, I will provide you with simple recipes and menus that take little time and do not require you to buy expensive products from the other side of the world. For example, try our simple and tasty One-Pot Chicken and Broccoli Stir Fry.

As a registered dietitian specializing in cardiovascular health for over ten years, I have helped numerous patients suffering from hypertension cope with their condition. I have often complemented my recommendations with practical advice and personal experiences. My interest in dietetics was inspired by the awareness of how well-thought-out changes in my family's diet helped my relatives effectively cope with chronic diseases. Therefore, I consider this cookbook, to be both the culmination of my professional path and my contribution to the creation of a healthy lifestyle.. It not only reduces your blood pressure, but also reduces the risk of heart disease, stroke, and diabetes. Rather than only improving your physical health, this diet plan will also develop your mind and strengthen you, causing you to be completely pleased. In this book, you will find how minimal steps right now can create fantastic outcomes and last a lengthy time.

The effectiveness of the Diet Approach to Stop Hypertension diet has been well studied and the results are convincing. There is ample evidence to support DASH's ability to control and reduce high blood pressure. Recent research gathered from a survey of the readers of previous DASH guides illustrates the above statement very vividly. Specifically, the survey found that 85% of respondents had checked and noticed reduced blood pressure within two months of strict adherence to the diet and incorporation of all the recommended foods. Beyond the reduction in blood pressure, the participants also experienced increased energy levels and decreased stress; when these factors come together, they contribute to well-being and a better quality of life. As a result, the research findings boost the confidence of the target participants as they consider adopting this change. Furthermore, the additional health benefits serve as evidence that the DASH diet takes an approach to promoting good health. This type of diet does not just focus on heart health; it also ensures well-being across other aspects of health and lifestyle. The above account has an impact that would be beneficial for anyone seeking to enhance their health and enjoy a better lifestyle.

This book is fully committed to assisting you in understanding the DASH diet completely and adopting it into your life satisfactorily and for the long-term. It is more than just a guide of dietary lists; it is a pathway to shifting your lifestyle to a better health opportunity. With creative, resourceful recipes and a graph of planned meals, you will undoubtedly be guaranteed not just to follow a food catalog but to significantly improve your livelihood. It is a one-stop guide to comprehending how to handle hypertension and improve your health while eating to your satisfaction. With this book, you are committing to a journey of a lifetime of better living through food. With a guide of this nature, you can adopt changes that will last and become your everyday processes.

This cookbook gives you a complete overview of the DASH diet, including its health benefits. It contains 150 healthy and delicious DASH-diet recipes that come from different categories, from breakfast to desserts. All the recipes in this cookbook are authentic and written with their exact preparation and cooking time, followed by step-by-step instructions, ending with their nutritional value information. This helps to keep track of your daily calorie intake. Thanks for choosing my cookbook. I hope you love and enjoy all the DASH-diet recipes written in this cookbook.

The DASH diet evolves dietary approaches to stop hypertension. It is one of the properly designed nutrition plans specifically intended to solve high blood pressure, a prevalent illness worldwide. Based on studies to manage hypertension, this diet is known for reducing blood pressure and improving general cardiovascular health. The DASH diet encourages the consumption of a wide range of fruits, vegetables, and low-fat dairy foods while eating mostly whole grains, fish, poultry, and nuts. Unlike anything else, it excessively lowers saturated fats, cholesterol, and refined sugar due to limiting red meat, sweets, and other heavy-fat products.

The DASH diet focuses on elements including the following:

Whole Grains: Whole grains are loaded with high fiber content that helps aid in heart health improvement and also maintain control over blood sugar levels.

Fruits and Vegetables: These play an important role by providing essential nutrients such as vitamins, minerals, and fibers that help in lowering blood pressure levels.

Dairy fats: Dairy fats are highlighted for their richness of calcium, protein, and vitamin D content. The dairy products used in the DASH diet are mostly low in fat.

Lean Proteins: Options such as poultry, fish, and legumes are preferred due to their fat levels compared to red meats.

Nuts and Legumes: Nuts and legumes are included for their healthy fats which can help to reduce bad cholesterol levels and promote a healthy heart.

The diet insists on limiting sodium as well as increasing potassium, calcium, and magnesium intake from food rather than supplements. This approach to nutrients not only allows you to reduce blood pressure levels but also to protect yourself from osteoporosis, cancer, heart disease, stroke, and diabetes.

DASH diet adherents are recommended to gradually increase fruits and vegetables and gradually include dairy through adaptation of the digestive system. As it can take many forms, the DASH diet is appropriate not only for patients with hypertension but also for people who simply strive to maintain a healthy lifestyle.

The Dietary Approaches to Stop Hypertension diet is one of the healthiest and most beneficial diet plans. Hence, the diet is well-studied for its potential to help fight hypertension. Hypertension is one of the main contributing factors in developing heart disease and stroke. Having been developed by research sponsored by the U.S. National Institutes of Health, the DASH diet is not only effective for pressure control but also useful for other health issues:

1. **Reduce blood pressure:** Although the DASH diet was first developed to help regulate blood pressure, it has been found to lower blood pressure effectively. In as little as two weeks, the diet redresses the imbalance between purging and eating meals that are abundant in potassium, calcium, or magnesium substances that can help reduce blood pressure.

2. **Heart-healthy diet:** The DASH eating plan supports heart health by its makeup. It contains fats, such as saturated and trans fats, and includes plenty of whole grains, fruits, and vegetables. These food selections play a role in lowering LDL cholesterol levels, which are closely linked to heart issues.

3. **Weight management:** The high fiber content resulting from eating the right proportions makes the DASH diet a viable way to lose weight and stay within an ideal range. Foods with a lot of fiber should help you glut your belly for a more extended period, and thus no or fewer hunger pangs should be felt. Since hunger management is crucial for good weight control, the DASH diet is important because it provides a practical method.

4. **Diabetes control and prevention:** The DASH diet reduces the risk of developing these problems, and provides the ability to manage them effectively, as the general balanced food focus is on nutrient-rich foods with a low glycemic index eaten in moderate quantities. Ensuring that the body receives the appropriate amount of carbs and proteins, as well as the preferred intake of fats, are critical aspects of controlling blood sugar levels. However, principles such as consuming as much food from these food groups as feasible, or portion sizes, may be followed in order to promote better control of glucose, which is crucial for preventing diabetes from developing and managing the disease. In general, studies show that whole, unprocessed foods are superior for moderating metabolic health and preventing the first warning signs and symptoms of diabetes.

5. **Reduce risk of developing cancer:** Research has suggested that the DASH eating pattern with its high content of fruits, vegetables, and fiber-containing foods may help to reduce the risk of certain cancers, such as colorectal and breast cancer. This protective benefit is likely to be mediated by the antioxidants and phytochemicals in these foods and amplifies the potential of a DASH-style diet to minimize cancer.

6. **Improves bone health:** The DASH diet improves bone health with the choice of dairy products that are rich in calcium and other magnesium and potassium-containing foods. Blessed with essential minerals, the DASH diet helps to support optimal bone density and protect from osteoporosis and other diseases. Regardless of disease treatment, this diet is beneficial, because strong bones affect the quality of your life. It is evident that calcium, magnesium, and potassium work with a balancing effect in preventing bone disorders.

7. **Longevity:** The longevity of the DASH diet is likely to add years to your life by reducing the presence of risk factors for chronic diseases and promoting a healthier way of living. The diet in question decreases the chances of developing conditions such as hypertension, heart disease, and diabetes, among other factors that traditionally result in the ultimate shortening of lifespan. Additionally, the diet is balanced and rich in nutrients; when consumed regularly and in proper quantities, it can ensure good health and may lead to a longer lifespan.

8. **Improved Mental Health:** Research has begun to demonstrate a correlation between diet and mental health. Nutrient-dense eating habits such as the DASH diet, which is abundant with fruits, vegetables, whole grains, and fish, has been shown to decrease the risk of depression and elevate general well-being.

9. **Anti-Inflammatory:** The DASH diet's anti-inflammatory advantages can be attributed to the large number of antioxidants in fruits, vegetables, nuts, and whole grains. Chronic inflammation is the root of numerous dangerous diseases such as cardiac disease, type-2 diabetes, and rheumatoid arthritis.

Overall, the DASH diet is a complete program that improves not only blood pressure but also the cardiovascular system, helps control weight, supports mental health, reduces the risk of cancer, and prolongs life. Being oriented on well-being throughout life, it is suitable for any person who cares about improving their quality of life, not just people with hypertension.

The DASH diet is one of the diets that are highly acknowledged for reducing blood pressure and enhancing cardiovascular health. As presented in my book, this diet aims to promote a balanced, healthy eating pattern by integrating foods with high nutrient content, such as fiber, lean protein, and critical minerals. In addition, the consumption of sodium, saturated fats, and added sugars should be kept to a minimum. This guide illustrates key components and fundamental items required in the basic DASH diet. The food groups include a wide selection that promotes a balanced diet and nutritional intake.

1. **Fruits and vegetables:**
   Fruits and vegetables are good sources of vitamins, minerals, fiber, and antioxidants, which are essential to the DASH diet.
   Leafy greens: Leafy greens such as spinach, kale, and Swiss chard are rich sources of potassium and magnesium. They help to improve heart functions.
   Cruciferous vegetables: Brussels sprouts, cauliflower, and broccoli contain healthy fiber and phytonutrients that assist in reducing inflammation.
   Fruits: Dark-colored fruits such as apples, oranges, and berries are rich in vitamin C and dietary fiber, which are required to boost your immunity and vascular health.

2. **Whole grains:**
   Whole grains are among the prolonged energy sources for the body. They are also great sources of fiber which plays an important role in maintaining cholesterol levels.
   Quinoa and Farro: These grains come with great protein and fiber content which are prime alternatives for refined carbohydrates.
   Whole wheat: It contains more nutrients and fiber compared to its refined form. Wheat should be used in baking and making pasta.
   Oats: They are best known for their beta-glucan fiber which help to lower cholesterol levels drastically.

3. **Proteins:**
   For those who want to lose weight, including lean sources of protein will help not only to cope with hunger but also to retain muscle.
   Fish: For example, salmon, mackerel, and brown trout are high in Omega-3 fatty acids.
   Poultry: Skinless chicken and turkey are low-fat products.
   Legumes: Beans, lentils, and chickpeas are not only good protein sources but also rich in fiber and minerals.

4. **Dairy**
   Low-fat and non-fat dairy products provide good amounts of calcium without the excessive saturated fat.
   Milk: Instead of choosing whole milk, which packs on fat, consider skim or 1% milk to reduce fat intake. Importantly, this does not come with a drop in calcium.

Yogurt and cheese: Low-fat yogurt and cheese do more than increase calcium intake; they also limit fat consumption.

5. **Nuts, seeds, and legumes**

   Nuts and seeds are good energy, protein, and fiber sources. They also provide essential fatty acids and magnesium.

   Almonds, walnuts, and pistachios: These are rich in monounsaturated fats.

   Flaxseeds and chia seeds: These are high in Omega-3 fatty acids.

   Peas and beans: Fiber and protein intake is achieved through eating peas and beans.

6. **Fat and oil**

   Fat is also necessary for a heart-healthy diet but should be consumed in moderation. It is important to choose the right fats.

   Olive oil: Is rich in heart-healthy mono-unsaturated fats.

   Canola oil: Contains less saturated fat and more mono- and polyunsaturated fats.

   Avocado: A source of beneficial fats that creates the same feeling of cream and tenderness in food, but with healthier fats.

7. **Spices**

   Spices can add flavor without extra salt, which makes blood pressure easier to control.

   Garlic and onions: They are bold and have the potential to lower cholesterol levels.

   Turmeric and cinnamon: They are anti-inflammatory.

   Basil, rosemary, and thyme: They can add flavor while maintaining salt levels.

8. **Beverages**

   Consider not just what you eat but also the importance of what drinks you put in your mouth.

   Water: Hydrating and is essential for normal cell activity.

   Green tea: Antioxidants for heart work.

   Low-sodium veggie juice: Easy and quick way to consume vegetables.

9. **Pantry Storage**

   Having the items below in your pantry makes cooking easier for you as you are likely to use the right DASH ingredients.

   Canned tomatoes: Buy a nutrient-rich soup or stew seasoned with canned tomatoes with low acidity.

   Whole grain flour: A staple supplement in breads and other grain goods.

   Low-sodium broth or stock: Prepare your own from home and use it carefully to make soups and stews.

NON-COMPATIBLE FOOD GROUPS: Limit non-compliant foods. To better follow the DASH diet, there are important things to limit:

1) **Sugary items:** Keep a low intake of candies, cookies, and other desserts.

2) **Red or meat too dense:** Some meat, including but not limited to red meat, are unduly dense; instead, it is better to choose fish or poultry.

3) **Fat content:** Avoid trans fats and limit your saturated fats intake.

Here are some tips to help you start the DASH diet:

1. Learn the food groups

When on the DASH diet, it is essential to understand which foods the diet emphasizes. The following is recommended in terms of servings to have each day:

Fruits and Vegetables: **4 to 5** servings per day.

Whole Grain: **6 to 8** servings per day.

Lean Protein: Choose **2 or fewer** servings of lean meats, poultry, and fish per day.

Dairy: **2 to 3** servings of low-fat or non-fat dairy per day.

Nuts, Seeds, and Legumes: **4 to 5** servings per week.

Fats and Oils: **2 to 3** healthy fat servings per day.

2. Add more vegetables and fruits to your meals

In addition to adding crucial vitamins and minerals to your diet, adding additional vegetables and fruits can be advantageous since it can boost your fiber consumption, which promotes digestion and heart health. Both freshly picked and frozen or tinned varieties are excellent alternatives, as long as they are not full of added sugars or salt.

3. Keep it simple with grains; choose whole grains

White bread and pasta may be replaced with whole grains in your meal. Whole grains are rich in vitamins and fibers, which are required for a healthy heart and stomach fullness.

4. Always choose low-fat dairy foods

When consuming low-fat or fat-free dairy products, you may receive your calcium, potassium, and vitamin D without consuming saturated fats.

5. Reduce your daily sodium intake

The DASH-diet element of eating or drinking low sodium is essential for lowering blood pressure. Most canned, processed, or high-sodium foods should be avoided entirely, such as cooked foods, fast foods, and processed products, among many others. Use a variety of spices or herbs instead of salt for flavor.

6. Include lean proteins

Your protein sources should be fish, poultry, and legumes. You should also reserve red meat for no more than twice a week and choose lean cuts to limit saturated fat consumption.

7. Include healthy fats

Consume healthy fats present in olive oil, avocados, and various nuts. These fats can help make blood cholesterol levels better while providing fats necessary for the body to run smoothly.

8. Plan Your Meals

Meal planning may guide you through the DASH diet. When doing your daily meal plans, ensure that you incorporate recommended foods from each food group for the week. This way, you will not only create a nutritional balance, but you will also reduce monotony in your diet.

9. Read Food Labels

Be more conscious of food labeling to gain more information on the food you eat. Pay attention to sodium levels, sugars, and fats.

10. Stay hydrated

Hydration is essential for general health and may help reduce hunger and ensure good digestion. Try drinking more fluids, preferably water.

11. Consult your doctor before starting any diet

Before starting any new diet, particularly if you have any health conditions, first consult your doctor or dietitian who can give you a plan as per your health conditions.

1-Blueberry Oatmeal

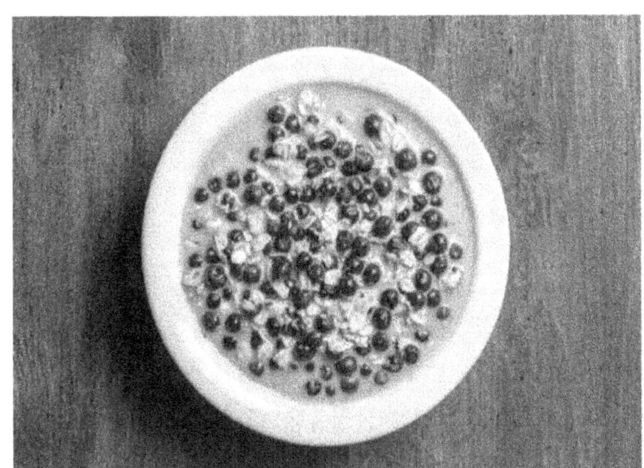

Preparation Time: 10 minutes
Cooking Time: 5 minutes
Serves: 1
Ingredients:

- ½ cup old-fashioned oats
- 2 tbsp unsweetened almond milk
- ½ cup blueberries
- ¼ tsp cinnamon
- ¼ tsp ground ginger
- 1 cup water
- 2 tbsp almonds, roasted & chopped

Directions:

Add water to a small saucepan and bring to a simmer over high heat. Add oatmeal, then turn heat to medium and cook oatmeal for 5 minutes.

Stir in blueberries, cinnamon, and ginger. Turn heat to low and cook until the blueberries are warm. Remove saucepan from heat.

Add almond milk and stir everything well.

Transfer oatmeal to a serving bowl and top with chopped almonds.

Serve and enjoy.

Nutritional Data: 261 calories | 63.61g carbs | 5.33g fat | 9.73g protein | 32mg sodium

2-Avocado Toast

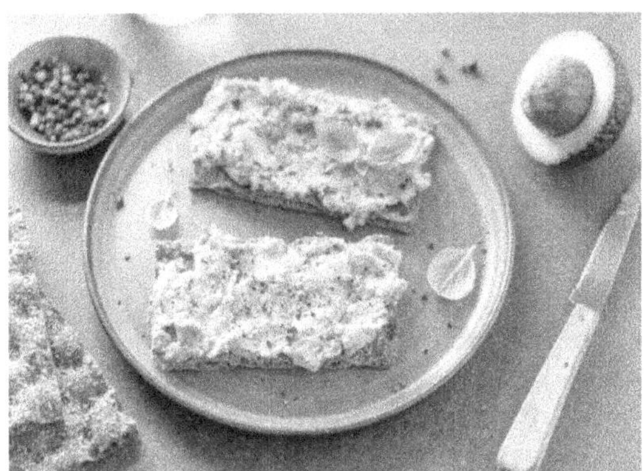

Preparation Time: 5 minutes
Cooking Time: 5 minutes
Serves: 2
Ingredients:

- 1 avocado, flesh scooped out
- 2 whole grain bread slices
- ½ tsp olive oil
- ½ tbsp fresh cilantro, chopped
- ¼ tsp red pepper flakes, crushed
- 2 tbsp onion, chopped
- 2 tsp lemon juice
- ¼ tsp garlic powder

Directions:

Add avocado flesh to a bowl and mash using a fork. Add garlic powder and lemon juice and mix well.

Toast bread slices in a pan over medium heat with olive oil.

Spread the avocado mixture on top of the bread slices. Garnish it with red pepper flakes, cilantro, and onions.

Serve and enjoy.

Nutritional Data: 288 calories | 28.46g carbs | 17.66g fat | 7.8g protein | 164mg sodium

3-Greek Yogurt Parfait

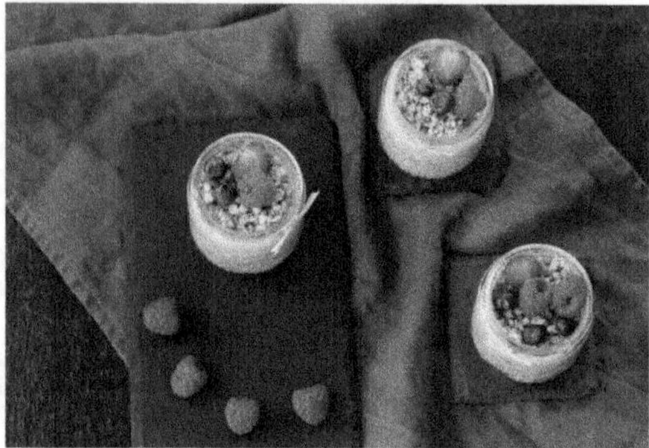

Preparation Time: 10 minutes
Cooking Time: 15 minutes
Serves: 1
Ingredients:

- ¾ cup Greek yogurt
- ¼ cup blueberries
- ¼ cup raspberries
- 1 tsp coconut oil, melted
- 1 tsp honey
- ½ tbsp sunflower seeds
- ½ tbsp pumpkin seeds
- 2 tbsp rolled oats

Directions:

Preheat the oven to 350° F.

Line baking sheet with parchment paper and set aside.

In a small bowl, mix oats, pumpkin seeds, sunflower seeds, honey, and melted coconut oil.

Spread the oat mixture onto a prepared baking sheet and bake in preheated oven for 15 minutes. Stir halfway through. Remove oat mixture from oven and let it cool completely.

Pour half of the yogurt into a mason jar, then add half of the oat mixture, then add half of the berries.

Add remaining yogurt and berries on top.

Serve and enjoy.

Nutritional Data: 359 calories | 50.78g carbs | 10.41g fat | 23.78g protein | 81mg sodium

4-Veggie Omelet

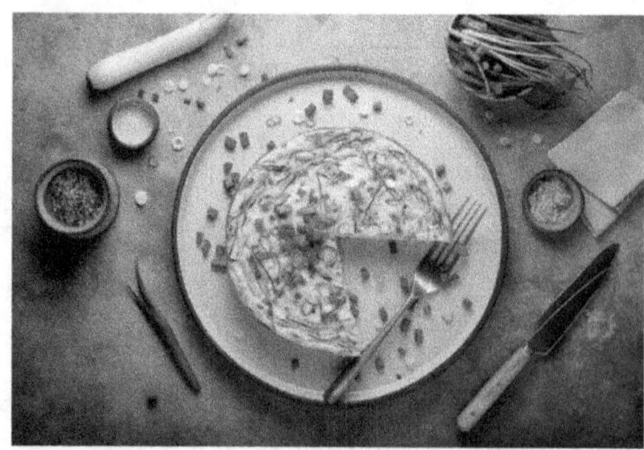

Preparation Time: 10 minutes
Cooking Time: 35 minutes
Serves: 6
Ingredients:

- 10 eggs
- 3 tbsp unsweetened almond milk
- 1 ½ cups cheddar cheese, shredded
- 1 cup fresh spinach, chopped
- 1 cup red pepper, chopped
- 2 tomatoes, chopped
- 1 small onion, chopped
- ½ tsp pepper

Directions:

Preheat the oven to 375° F.

In a mixing bowl, whisk eggs with almond milk and pepper. Add 1 cup cheddar cheese, spinach, red pepper, tomatoes, and onion, and mix everything well.

Pour the egg mixture into the greased casserole dish and top with remaining shredded cheese.

Bake in preheated oven for 35 minutes.

Slice and serve.

Nutritional Data: 342 calories | 12.82g carbs | 21.54g fat | 23.72g protein | 830mg sodium

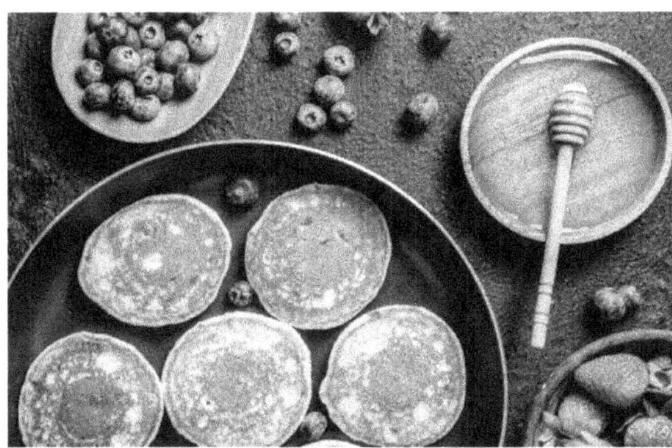

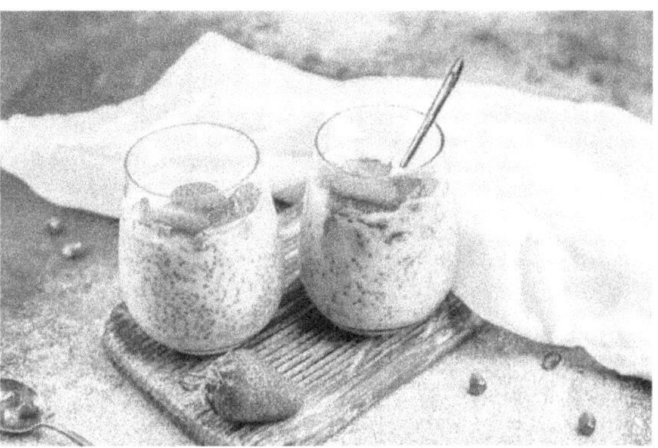

Preparation Time: 10 minutes
Cooking Time: 15 minutes
Serves: 8
Ingredients:

- 2 eggs
- 2 cups whole wheat flour
- 2 tbsp canola oil
- 1 ½ cups buttermilk
- 4 tsp baking powder

Directions:

In a small bowl, mix together flour and baking powder.

In a separate bowl, whisk together eggs, canola oil, and buttermilk. Add flour mixture and mix until just combined.

Lightly grease a pan with cooking spray and heat over medium heat for 30 seconds.

Pour a spoonful of batter onto the hot pan and cook until lightly golden brown on both sides.

Serve and enjoy.

Nutritional Data: 186 calories | 25.22g carbs | 7.07g fat | 7.73g protein | 116mg sodium

Preparation Time: 5 minutes
Cooking Time: 5 minutes
Serves: 2
Ingredients:

- ¼ cup chia seeds
- 1 tsp vanilla extract
- 2 tbsp honey
- 1 cup unsweetened almond milk
- ¼ cup fresh berries

Directions:

In a bowl, whisk together almond milk, vanilla, and honey until combined. Add chia seeds and stir well.

Transfer the chia seed mixture into two serving glass jars. Cover the jar with lids and place it in the refrigerator overnight.

Top with fresh berries and serve.

Nutritional Data: 314 calories | 51.04g carbs | 10.76g fat | 5.71g protein | 145mg sodium

7-Banana Smoothie

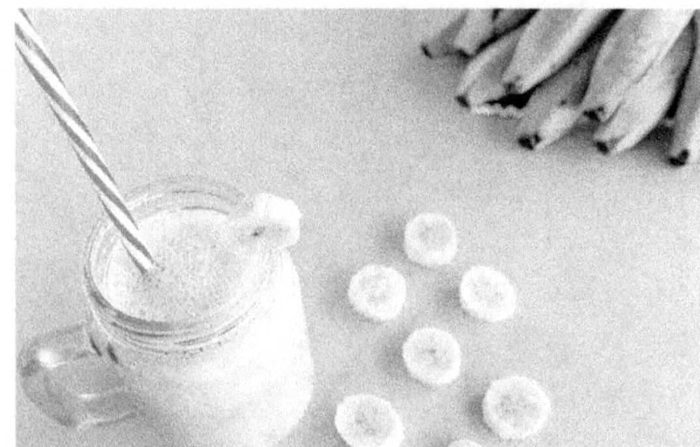

Preparation Time: 5 minutes
Cooking Time: 5 minutes
Serves: 2
Ingredients:

- 1 large banana
- Pinch of cinnamon
- 4 ice cubes
- 1 tsp vanilla
- 2 tbsp chia seeds
- 2 tbsp sunflower seeds
- ¼ cup walnuts
- ¼ cup almonds
- 1 cup unsweetened almond milk
- 4 dates, pitted

Directions:

Add banana and remaining ingredients into the blender and blend until smooth.

Pour the smoothie into two serving glasses.

Serve immediately and enjoy.

Nutritional Data: 334 calories | 45.48g carbs | 15.96g fat | 6.89g protein | 89mg sodium

8-Egg and Spinach Breakfast Wrap

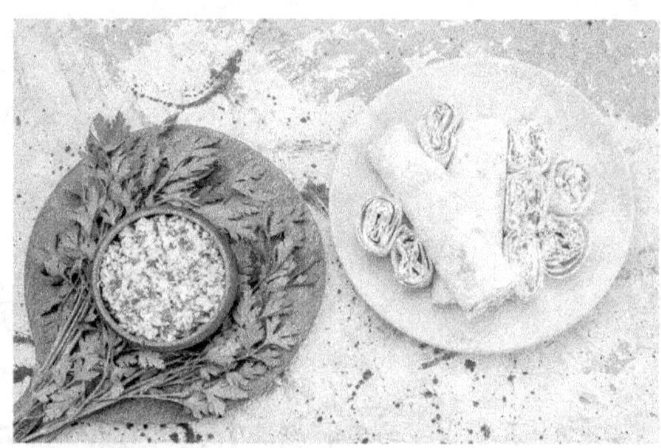

Preparation Time: 10 minutes
Cooking Time: 10 minutes
Serves: 1
Ingredients:

- 1 egg
- ¼ cup egg whites
- 1 whole grain tortilla
- 1 tbsp sun-dried tomatoes, chopped
- 1 tbsp feta cheese, crumbled
- 2 cups baby spinach
- 2 mushrooms, sliced
- 2 tbsp hummus
- 2 tbsp onion, chopped
- Pepper

Directions:

Spray pan with cooking spray and sauté mushrooms and onion over medium heat for 2–4 minutes. Add spinach and sauté until spinach is wilted.

Add egg whites and egg to pan with veggies and cook for 2–3 minutes. Season with pepper.

Warm up the tortilla in a pan. Spread hummus over tortilla then add veggie-egg mixture in the center of the tortilla and top with feta cheese and sun-dried tomatoes.

Wrap tortilla and serve.

Nutritional Data: 746 calories | 42.21g carbs | 45.35g fat | 45.36g protein | 1712mg sodium

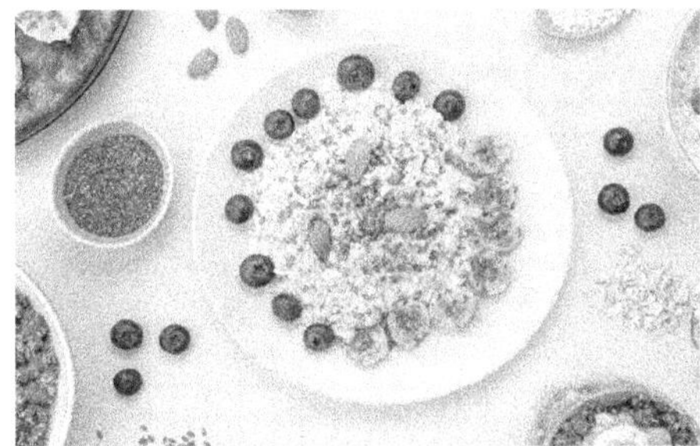

Preparation Time: 10 minutes
Cooking Time: 15 minutes
Serves: 2
Ingredients:

- ½ cup quinoa, rinsed & drained
- 1 tbsp almond butter
- 2 tbsp raisins
- ½ tbsp chia seeds
- ½ tsp vanilla
- 1 tsp cinnamon
- 1 cup unsweetened almond milk

Directions:

Add quinoa, almond milk, cinnamon, and vanilla in a small saucepan and bring to a boil.

Turn heat to low and simmer for 15 minutes or until all liquid is absorbed.

Transfer quinoa into a bowl and top with almond butter, raisins, and chia seeds.

Serve and enjoy.

Nutritional Data: 334 calories | 46.87g carbs | 12.38g fat | 10.57g protein | 108mg sodium

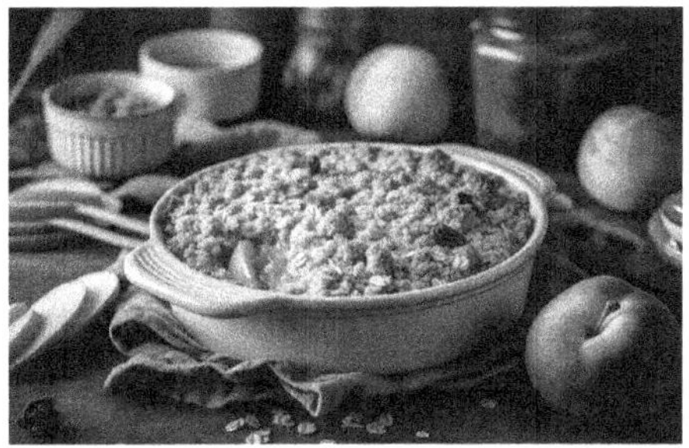

Preparation Time: 10 minutes
Cooking Time: 30 minutes
Serves: 9
Ingredients:

- 2 cups apples, chopped
- 1 tsp baking powder
- ¼ tsp ground allspice
- ¼ tsp ground cloves
- ¼ tsp ground nutmeg
- 2 tsp ground cinnamon
- 2 cups rolled oats
- 2 bananas
- 2 tsp vanilla
- 1 ¾ cups unsweetened almond milk

Directions:

Preheat the oven to 350° F.

In a mixing bowl, add bananas and mash using a fork. Add almond milk and vanilla and mix well.

In a separate bowl, mix oats, baking powder, allspice, cloves, nutmeg, and cinnamon.

Pour banana mixture over oat mixture and mix until just combined.

Add 1 ½ cups of chopped apples and fold well.

Pour batter into the 9x9-inch greased baking dish. Spread the remaining chopped apples on top.

Cover the baking dish with foil and bake in preheated oven for 20 minutes. Remove foil and bake for 10 minutes more.

Slice and serve.

Nutritional Data: 746 calories | 42.21g carbs | 45.35g fat | 45.36g protein | 1712mg sodium

11-Ricotta & Berry Toast

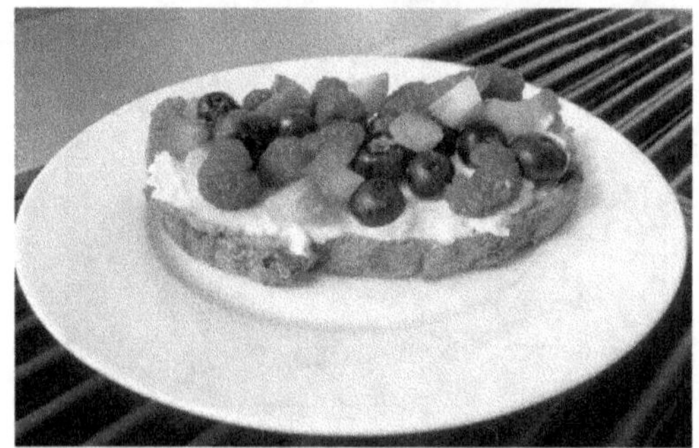

Preparation Time: 5 minutes
Cooking Time: 5 minutes
Serves: 2
Ingredients:
- 2 whole grain bread slices, toasted
- ½ cup fresh mixed berries
- ½ tsp lemon zest, grated
- 2 tsp maple syrup
- ¼ cup ricotta cheese

Directions:

In a small bowl, mix ricotta cheese, lemon zest, and maple syrup.

Spread the ricotta cheese mixture onto one side of each bread slice.

Top each toast with mixed berries and serve.

Nutritional Data: 352 calories | 49.67g carbs | 10.5g fat | 14.9g protein | 384mg sodium

12-Sweet Potato Hash

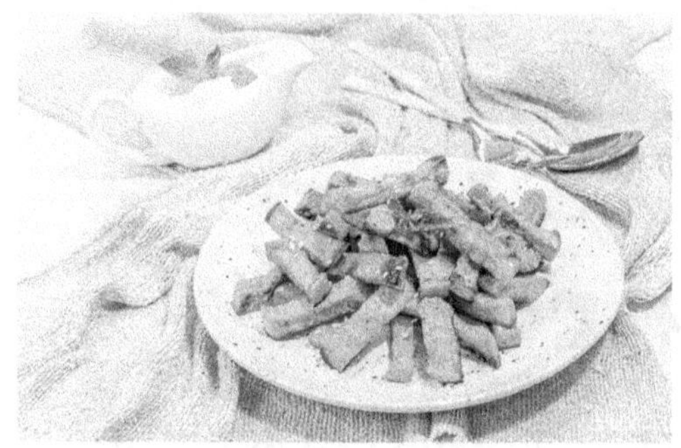

Preparation Time: 10 minutes
Cooking Time: 20 minutes
Serves: 4
Ingredients:
- 1 lb sweet potatoes, cubed
- ¼ tsp pepper
- ½ green bell pepper, chopped
- ½ red bell pepper, chopped
- ½ onion, chopped
- 2 garlic cloves, chopped
- 2 tbsp olive oil

Directions:

Heat olive oil in a pan over medium heat.

Add sweet potato cubes to the pan, cover the pan, and cook over medium heat for 10 minutes. Stir occasionally.

Add remaining ingredients to the pan and stir well, cook for 10 minutes more.

Serve and enjoy.

Nutritional Data: 121 calories | 13.11g carbs | 7.38g fat | 3.35g protein | 9mg sodium

13-Mediterranean Breakfast Bowl

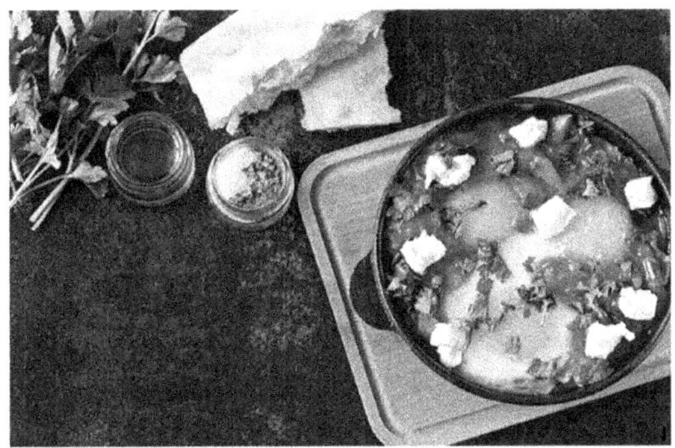

Preparation Time: 5 minutes
Cooking Time: 5 minutes
Serves: 1
Ingredients:

- 2 eggs
- 1 tsp olive oil
- ½ bell pepper, chopped
- ½ scallion, chopped
- ¼ cup olives, pitted
- ¼ cup feta cheese, crumbled
- Pepper

Directions:

Whisk eggs in a mixing bowl. Add olives, scallion, bell pepper, feta cheese, and pepper.

Heat oil in a pan over medium-high heat.

Add egg mixture and let cook for 2 minutes, then start scrambling the eggs for 3 minutes.

Serve and enjoy.

Nutritional Data: 466 calories | 12.6g carbs | 35.5g fat | 25.03g protein | 801mg sodium

14- Spinach and Mushroom Frittata

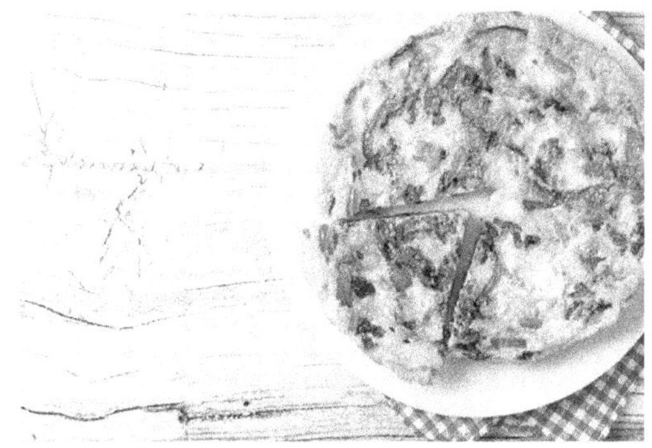

Preparation Time: 10 minutes
Cooking Time: 35 minutes
Serves: 4
Ingredients:

- 8 eggs
- 4 oz baby spinach
- 1 ½ tbsp olive oil
- 4 oz feta cheese, crumbled
- 2 tbsp plain yogurt
- ½ lb mushrooms, quartered
- 1 onion, sliced

Directions:

Preheat the oven to 400° F.

Heat oil in a skillet over medium heat.

Add onion and sauté for 5 minutes. Add mushrooms and cook until mushrooms soften, about 3–5 minutes.

Add spinach and cook until spinach is wilted. Remove pan from heat.

In a bowl, whisk eggs with yogurt. Add feta cheese and stir well.

Pour the egg mixture into the spinach-mushroom mixture and cook in preheated oven for 18–20 minutes.

Slice and serve.

Nutritional Data: 559 calories | 47.52g carbs | 31.31g fat | 28.5g protein | 498mg sodium

15-Peanut Butter Banana Smoothie

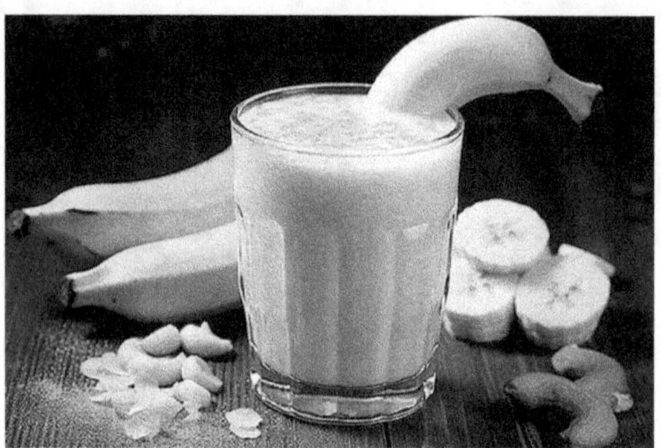

Preparation Time: 5 minutes
Cooking Time: 5 minutes
Serves: 2
Ingredients:

- ¼ cup peanut butter
- 2 cups banana
- 1 cup ice cubes
- 1 cup unsweetened almond milk
- ¼ cup Greek yogurt
- 2 tbsp honey

Directions:

Add peanut butter and remaining ingredients into the blender and blend until smooth.

Pour into the serving glasses and serve immediately.

Nutritional Data: 726 calories | 140.7g carbs | 17.6g fat | 12.64g protein | 615mg sodium

16-Oatmeal Banana Muffins

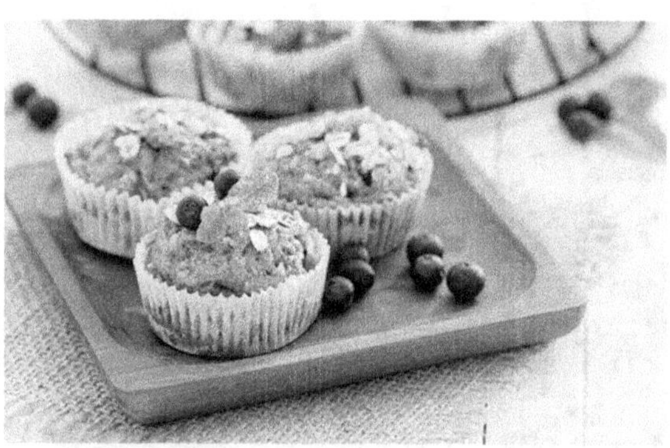

Preparation Time: 10 minutes
Cooking Time: 20 minutes
Serves: 12
Ingredients:

- 2 eggs
- 3 ripe bananas, mashed
- ½ tsp baking soda
- 1 tsp baking powder
- 1/8 tsp nutmeg
- 1 tsp cinnamon
- 1 ½ cups whole wheat flour
- 1 cup rolled oats
- ½ cup unsweetened almond milk
- ½ cup maple syrup

Directions:

Preheat the oven to 425° F.

Lightly grease muffin pan with cooking spray and set aside.

In a mixing bowl, add mashed bananas, eggs, milk, and maple syrup and mix until well combined.

Add oats and let sit for 5 minutes.

Add flour, baking soda, baking powder, and cinnamon and mix until just combined.

Spoon batter into the prepared muffin pan and bake in preheated oven for 15–20 minutes.

Serve and enjoy.

Nutritional Data: 165 calories | 31.73g carbs | 4.14g fat | 5.17g protein | 79mg sodium

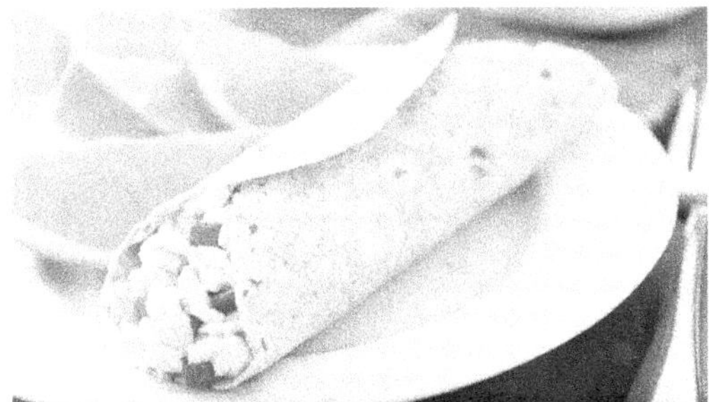

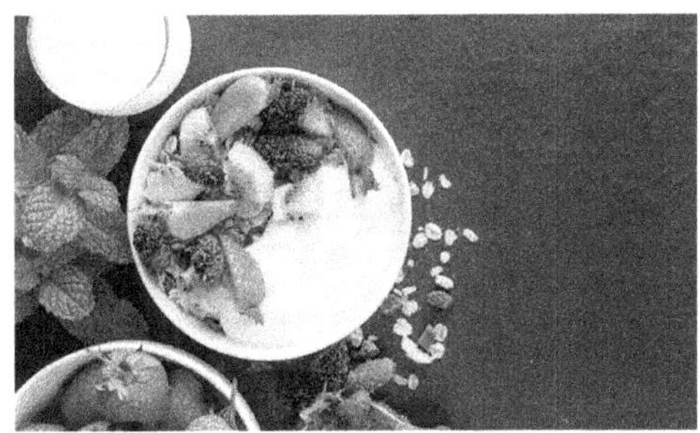

Preparation Time: 10 minutes
Cooking Time: 10 minutes
Serves: 4
Ingredients:

- 4 whole-wheat tortillas
- 8 eggs
- ½ cup low-fat cheddar cheese, shredded
- 1 tsp mixed herbs
- 3 tbsp unsweetened almond milk
- 1 cup spinach, chopped
- 1 zucchini, diced
- 1 bell pepper, diced
- 1 onion, diced
- 1 tbsp olive oil

Directions:

Heat ½ tablespoon of oil in a pan over medium heat.

Add onion and sauté for 4 minutes. Add zucchini and bell pepper and cook for 5 minutes or until veggies are softened.

Add spinach and cook until wilted. Remove pan from heat.

In a bowl, whisk eggs with mixed herbs and milk.

Pour the egg mixture into the separate pan and scramble until cooked.

Add scrambled eggs, sautéed veggies, and cheese in the middle of a tortilla.

Wrap tortilla and serve.

Nutritional Data: 726 calories | 140.7g carbs | 17.6g fat | 12.64g protein | 615mg sodium

Preparation Time: 5 minutes
Cooking Time: 5 minutes
Serves: 2
Ingredients:

- 1 cup cottage cheese
- ½ tbsp honey
- 1 tbsp mint leaves, chopped
- 1 tsp chia seeds
- ¼ cup blueberries
- ¼ cup raspberries
- ¼ cup blackberries
- 1 kiwi fruit, peeled & sliced
- 5 strawberries, sliced

Directions:

Divide cottage cheese into two serving bowls.

Top with fruit, mint, and chia seeds. Drizzle with honey.

Serve and enjoy.

Nutritional Data: 365 calories | 49.68g carbs | 12.54g fat | 17.21g protein | 392mg sodium

19-Pumpkin Spice Overnight Oats

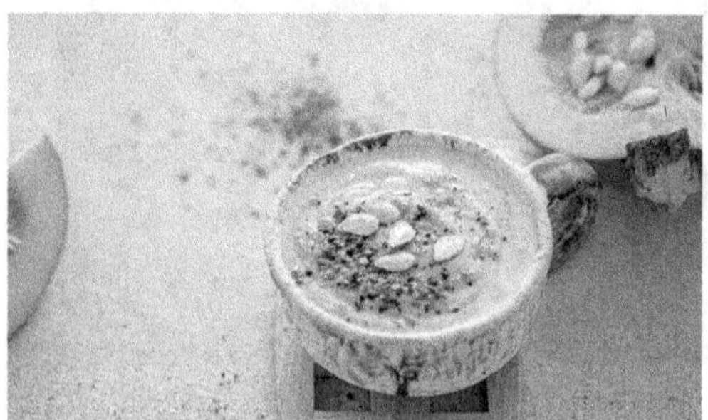

Preparation Time: 10 minutes
Cooking Time: 5 minutes
Serves: 4
Ingredients:

- 2 cups rolled oats
- 4 tsp chia seeds
- 2 tbsp maple syrup
- 1 tsp vanilla
- 2 tsp pumpkin spice
- ¼ cup pumpkin puree
- 2 cups unsweetened almond milk

Directions:

Divide oats and chia seeds into the four 8-ounce mason jars.

In a bowl, whisk almond milk, maple syrup, vanilla, pumpkin spice, and pumpkin puree until smooth, then pour equally into each jar.

Seal jar with lid, shake well, and place in refrigerator overnight.

Serve and enjoy.

Nutritional Data: 267 calories | 52.36g carbs | 9.61g fat | 11.72g protein | 108mg sodium

20-Turkey Sausage Breakfast Sandwich

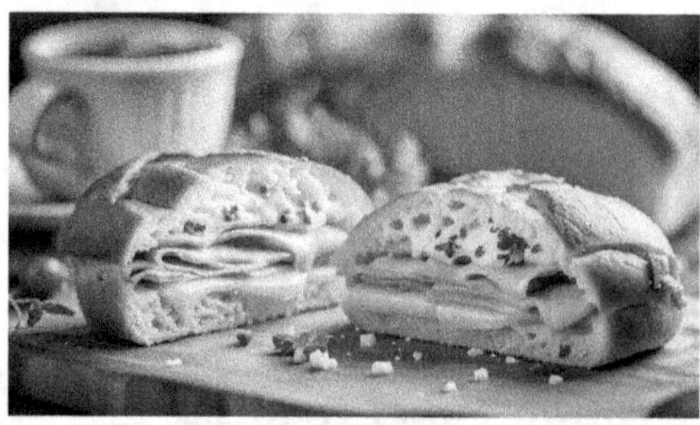

Preparation Time: 10 minutes
Cooking Time: 5 minutes
Serves: 1
Ingredients:

- 2 egg whites
- 1 whole-wheat English muffin, halved
- 1 cheddar cheese slice
- 1 turkey sausage patty

Directions:

Spray pan with cooking spray and heat over medium-low heat.

Add egg whites to pan and cook both sides. Remove pan from heat.

Heat the sausage patty in the microwave.

Toast the English muffin in the toaster.

Place cooked egg in toasted English muffin and top with cheddar cheese slice then add sausage patty and top with the other muffin half.

Serve and enjoy.

Nutritional Data: 360 calories | 27.92g carbs | 16.72g fat | 25:47g protein | 750mg sodium

21-Yogurt and Berry Smoothie Bowl

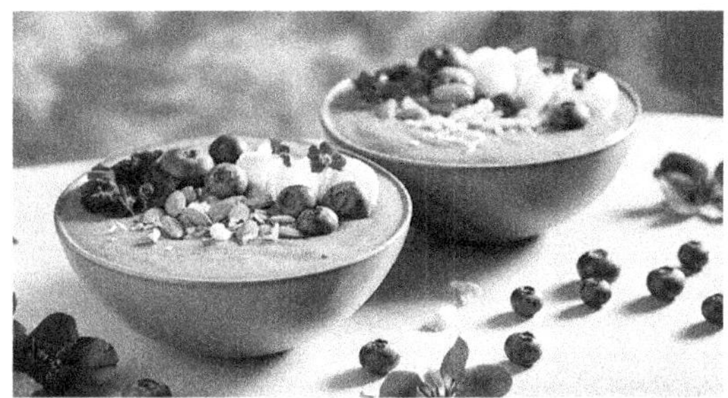

Preparation Time: 5 minutes
Cooking Time: 5 minutes
Serves: 2
Ingredients:

- 1 cup Greek yogurt
- 1 tsp honey
- ¼ cup water
- 1 tbsp chia seeds
- 1 tbsp almond butter
- 1 cup mixed berries

Directions:

Add yogurt and remaining ingredients into the blender and blend until smooth.

Pour the smoothie into serving bowls and top with your favorite toppings.

Serve and enjoy.

Nutritional Data: 429 calories | 59.32g carbs | 13.58g fat | 20.21g protein | 289mg sodium

22-Egg and Cheese Breakfast Quesadilla

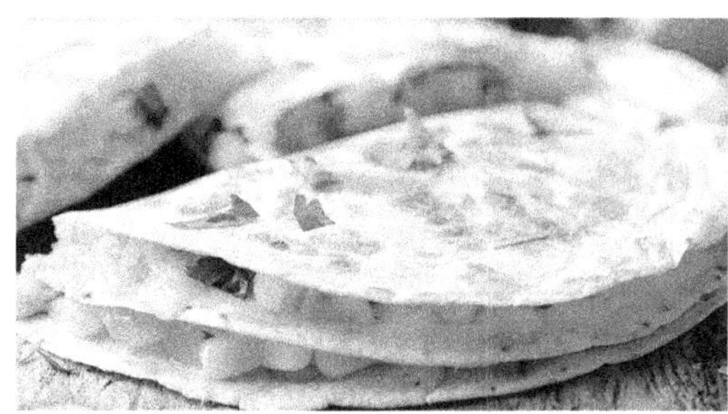

Preparation Time: 5 minutes
Cooking Time: 5 minutes
Serves: 1
Ingredients:

- 2 eggs
- 1/3 cup cheddar cheese, shredded
- 2 whole-wheat tortillas
- 2 tbsp olive oil

Directions:

Whisk eggs in a small bowl.

Heat 1 tablespoon of olive oil in a pan over medium heat. Add the eggs and cook until they are fluffy.

Once done, remove eggs from pan.

Heat 1/2 tablespoon of olive oil in a pan over medium heat.

Add one tortilla to the pan and top with a sprinkle of cheddar cheese.

Once the cheese is melted, add cooked eggs and spread evenly. Place the second tortilla on top.

Cook the tortilla until lightly brown on both sides.

Once it is brown, transfer the quesadilla to a cutting board and let it cool for 2 minutes.

Cut into triangle-shaped pieces and serve.

Nutritional Data: 889 calories | 48.01g carbs | 61.21g fat | 36.4g protein | 1484mg sodium

23-Almond Butter Banana Toast

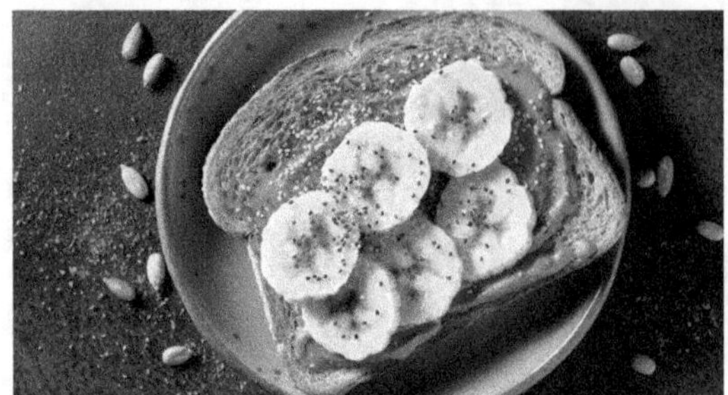

Preparation Time: 5 minutes
Cooking Time: 5 minutes
Serves: 2
Ingredients:

- 2 whole-wheat bread slices
- 1 banana, sliced
- 2 tbsp almond butter

Directions:

Place bread slices in a pan and toast them on medium heat.

Spread almond butter on toasted bread slices and top with sliced bananas.

Serve and enjoy

Nutritional Data: 297 calories | 46.74g carbs | 10.5g fat | 9.39g protein | 281mg sodium

24-Berry Quinoa Breakfast Bowl

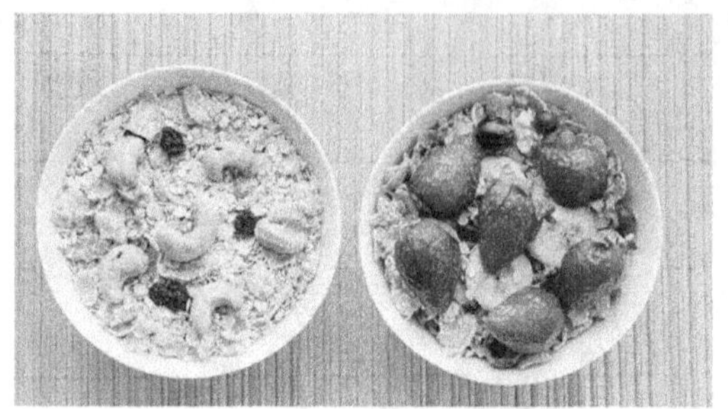

Preparation Time: 10 minutes
Cooking Time: 20 minutes
Serves: 2
Ingredients:

- ¼ cup quinoa, rinsed & drained
- ½ cup unsweetened almond milk
- 2 tsp hemp seeds
- ½ cup blueberries
- 5 strawberries, sliced
- ¼ cup raspberries
- 2 tsp honey
- ½ tsp vanilla
- ½ tsp cinnamon

Directions:

Add almond milk, vanilla, and cinnamon in a small saucepan and bring to a boil, reduce heat, and simmer.

Add quinoa, cover, and cook over low heat until liquid evaporates about 20 minutes.

Fluff quinoa with a fork.

Divide quinoa into two serving bowls. Top with hemp seeds and berries. Drizzle with honey.

Serve and enjoy.

Nutritional Data: 246 calories | 50.21g carbs | 3.88g fat | 4.91g protein | 48mg sodium

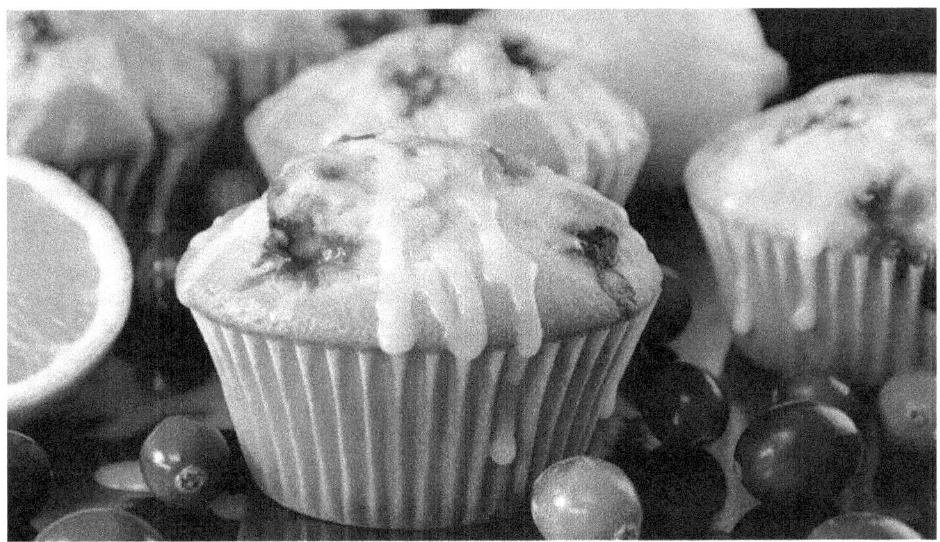

Preparation Time: 10 minutes
Cooking Time: 20 minutes
Serves: 12
Ingredients:

- 5 eggs
- 1 ½ tsp baking powder
- 1 tsp vanilla
- 1 tbsp orange zest
- ½ tsp cinnamon
- 3 tbsp butter, melted
- ¾ cup erythritol
- 3 tbsp heavy cream
- ¾ cup cranberries, chopped
- 2 tbsp coconut flour
- 2 cups almond flour

Directions:

Preheat the oven to 350° F.

Lightly grease the muffin pan with cooking spray and set aside.

In a mixing bowl, mix almond flour, baking powder, cinnamon, and coconut flour.

In a separate bowl, whisk eggs with butter, heavy cream, vanilla, erythritol, and orange zest until frothy.

Pour egg mixture into the almond flour mixture and mix until just combined.

Add cranberries and fold well.

Spoon batter into the prepared muffin pan and bake in preheated oven for 20 minutes.

Serve and enjoy.

Nutritional Data: 297 calories | 46.74g carbs | 10.5g fat | 9.39g protein | 281mg sodium

Chapter 3 — Appetizer Recipes

1-Greek Salad Skewers

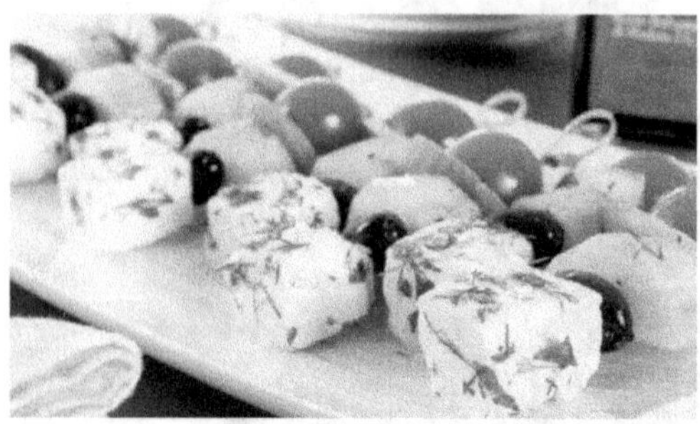

Preparation Time: 10 minutes
Cooking Time: 10 minutes
Serves: 24 skewers
Ingredients:

- 12 oz feta cheese, cut into small cubes
- 5 mini cucumbers, cut into ½-inch thick slices
- 24 olives, pitted
- 24 cherry tomatoes
- 1 tbsp lemon juice
- 1 tbsp dried oregano
- 1/3 cup olive oil
- Salt

Directions:

In a medium bowl, mix lemon juice, olive oil, oregano, and salt. Add feta cubes and mix until well coated. Cover and place in refrigerator for 2 hours to marinate.

On each wooden skewer, layer on a cherry tomato, olive, cucumber slice, and feta cube.

Serve immediately and enjoy.

Nutritional Data: 73 calories | 2.07g carbs | 6.42g fat | 2.14g protein | 172mg sodium

2-Hummus with Veggie Sticks

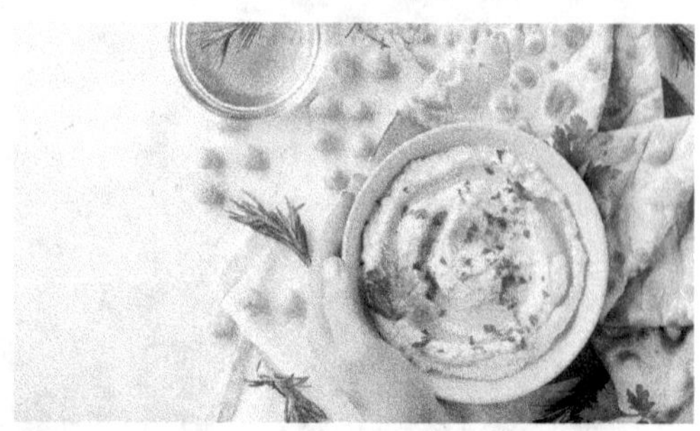

Preparation Time: 10 minutes
Cooking Time: 25 minutes
Serves: 4

- 28-oz can low-sodium chickpeas, drained & rinsed
- 2 garlic cloves
- 3 tbsp water
- ¼ tsp cumin
- 1 ½ tbsp lemon juice
- 1 tbsp tahini
- 2 tbsp olive oil
- Salt

Directions:

Add chickpeas and remaining ingredients into the food processor and process until smooth.

Serve hummus with vegetable sticks.

Nutritional Data: 360 calories | 47.13g carbs | 13.72g fat | 14.75g protein | 426mg sodium

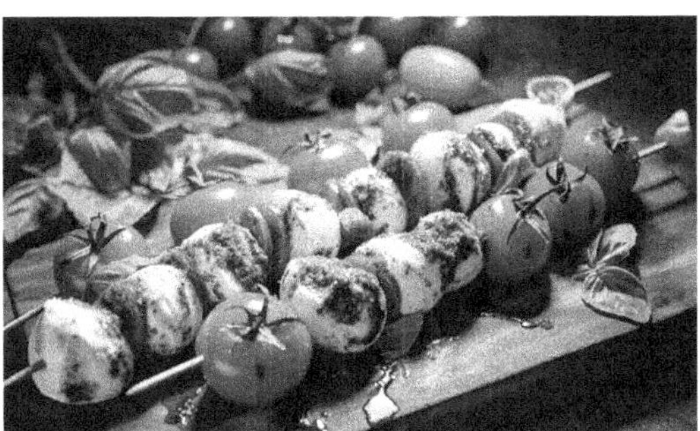

Preparation Time: 10 minutes
Cooking Time: 10 minutes
Serves: 24 skewers
Ingredients:

- 12 mini mozzarella balls
- 12 basil leaves
- 12 grape tomatoes
- 2 tsp balsamic vinegar
- 2 tbsp olive oil
- Pepper
- Salt

Directions:

Thread grape tomato, basil leaf, and mozzarella ball on each skewer.

In a small bowl, mix together vinegar, olive oil, pepper, and salt.

Drizzle vinegar mixture over skewers and serve.

Nutritional Data: 81 calories | 5.21g carbs | 6.84g fat | 0.5g protein | 6mg sodium

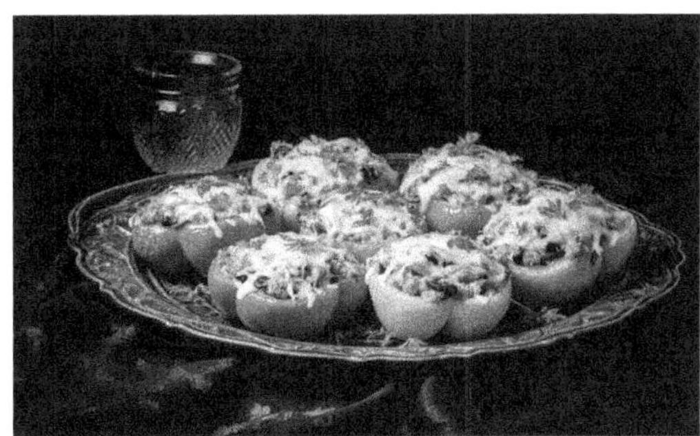

Preparation Time: 10 minutes
Cooking Time: 20 minutes
Serves: 8

- 8 mini bell peppers, cut lengthwise & seeds removed
- ¼ cup fresh cilantro, chopped
- 1 garlic clove, minced
- 2 tbsp olive oil
- 2 tbsp onion, diced
- 5 oz cream cheese
- Pepper
- Salt

Directions:

Preheat the oven to 350° F.

Line baking sheet with parchment paper and set aside.

Heat 1 tablespoon of oil in a pan over medium heat.

Add onion and sauté until softened. Add garlic and sauté for 1 minute.

Place mini peppers halved on the baking sheet and drizzle with remaining oil and cook in oven for 8 minutes.

In a small bowl, mix cream cheese, cilantro, garlic, onion, pepper, and salt.

Spoon the cream cheese mixture into the peppers and bake for 8 minutes more.

Serve and enjoy.

Nutritional Data: 177 calories | 4.21g carbs | 16.93g fat | 4.13g protein | 78mg sodium

5-Cucumber Avocado Sushi Rolls

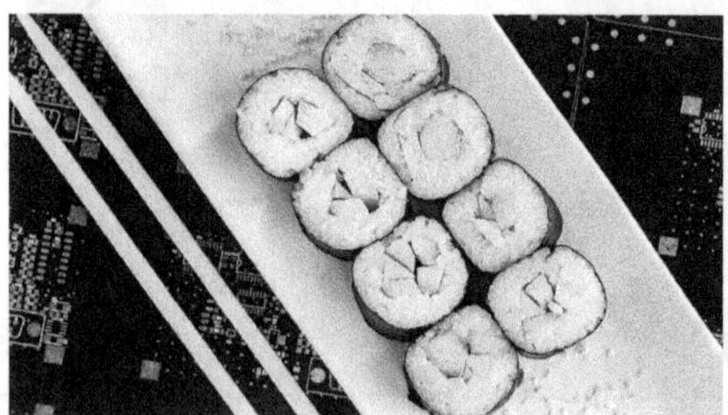

Preparation Time: 10 minutes
Cooking Time: 30 minutes
Serves: 6
Ingredients:

- 4 nori sheets
- 1 avocado, peeled and sliced
- 1/2 cucumber, sliced into thin strips
- 3 tbsp rice vinegar
- 1 cup sushi rice
- 1 1/2 cups water
- 1/8 tsp salt

Directions:

Add sushi rice, vinegar, water, and salt into the saucepan and bring to a boil. Reduce heat to low and simmer for 20 minutes. Remove from heat and set aside to cool.

Place a nori sheet on a bamboo mat and spread rice evenly on the nori.

Arrange cucumber and avocado slices on the rice layer.

Roll the nori sheet slowly around the ingredients until you reach the other end of the roll.

Cut the roll into slices and serve.

Nutritional Data: 117 calories | 12.71g carbs | 9.01g fat | 3.3g protein | 57mg sodium

6-Mediterranean Chickpea Salad Cups

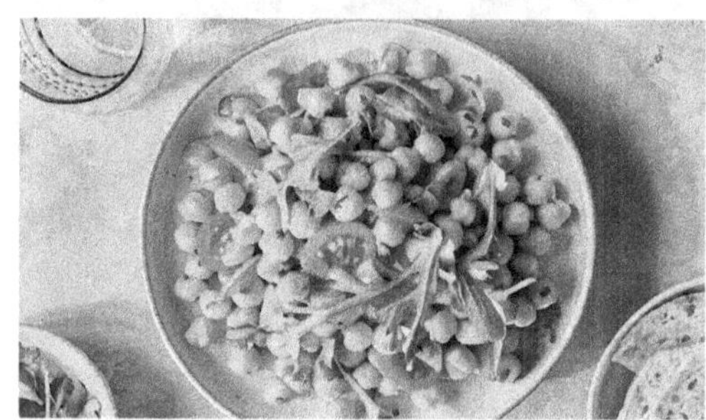

Preparation Time: 10 minutes
Cooking Time: 10 minutes
Serves: 6

- 15-oz can low-sodium chickpeas, drained & rinsed
- ¼ cup parsley, chopped
- ¼ cup sun-dried tomatoes, chopped
- ¼ tsp dried oregano
- 1 garlic clove, grated
- 3 tbsp olive oil
- 2 tbsp lemon juice
- 2 tbsp onion, diced
- Pepper
- Salt
- 6 Boston lettuce leaves

Directions:

In a mixing bowl, mix together chickpeas, parsley, sun-dried tomatoes, oregano, garlic, oil, lemon juice, onion, pepper, and salt.

Cover salad bowl and place in refrigerator for 15 minutes.

Add salad on lettuce leaves and serve.

Nutritional Data: 171 calories | 19.2g carbs | 8.62g fat | 5.62g protein | 158mg sodium

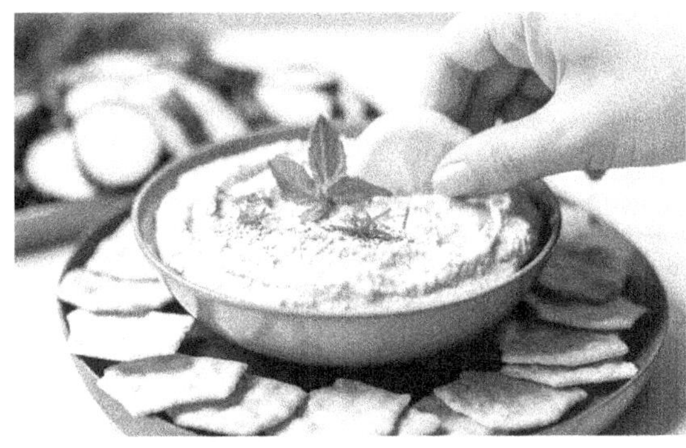

Preparation Time: 5 minutes
Cooking Time: 5 minutes
Serves: 6
Ingredients:

- 2 ¼ cups shelled edamame
- 4 tbsp water
- 2 garlic cloves, minced
- 3 tbsp olive oil
- ¼ cup lemon juice
- ¼ cup tahini
- Salt

Directions:

Add shelled edamame and remaining ingredients into the food processor and process until smooth and creamy.

Serve and enjoy.

Nutritional Data: 194 calories | 8.93g carbs | 15.18g fat | 8.12g protein | 60mg sodium

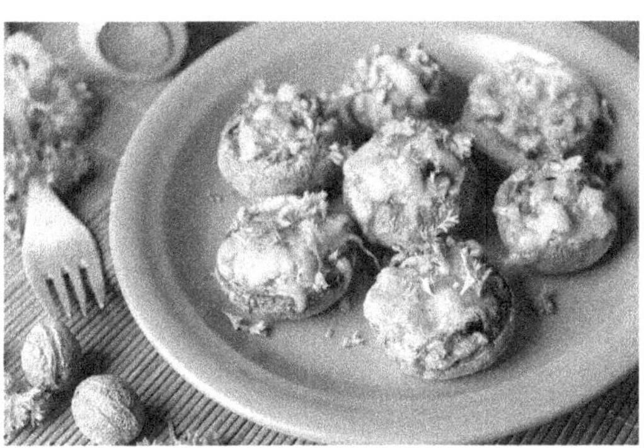

Preparation Time: 10 minutes
Cooking Time: 25 minutes
Serves: 4

- 12 mushrooms, cleaned & stems cut
- 1 tbsp olive oil
- 8 oz cream cheese
- ½ tsp paprika
- 2 tbsp fresh chives, chopped
- Pepper
- Salt

Directions:

Preheat the oven to 400° F.

Finely chop the mushroom stems.

Heat oil into pan over medium heat.

Add mushroom stems and sauté for 1 minute. Remove pan from heat.

In a bowl, mix together cream cheese, paprika, chives, sautéed mushroom stems, pepper, and salt.

Stuff cream cheese mixture into each mushroom.

Arrange mushrooms onto the baking dish and bake in preheated oven for 20 minutes.

Serve and enjoy.

Nutritional Data: 215 calories | 5.04g carbs | 19.85g fat | 6.01g protein | 251mg sodium

9-Tomato Basil Bruschetta

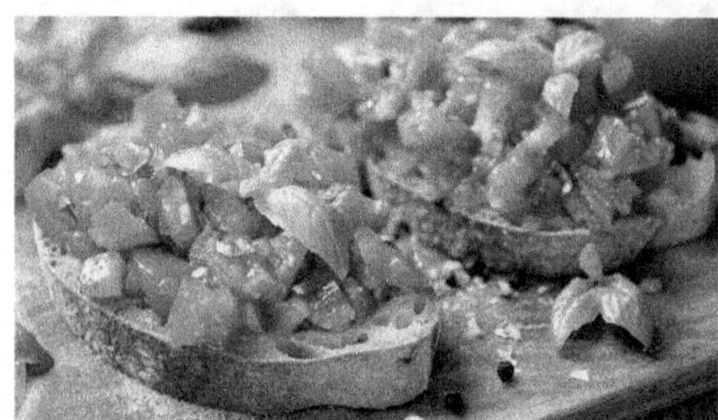

Preparation Time: 10 minutes
Cooking Time: 10 minutes
Serves: 4
Ingredients:

- 8 oz whole-wheat baguette bread, cut into 1-inch slices
- 2 tbsp garlic, minced
- 2 tbsp olive oil
- For topping:
- 4 oz mozzarella cheese, shredded
- 8 oz tomato, chopped
- 2 tsp honey
- 4 tbsp balsamic vinegar
- 0.5 oz basil, chopped
- 2 oz onions, chopped
- 1/8 tsp salt

Directions:

Preheat the Panini press.

In a small bowl, mix oil and garlic.

Brush bread slices with oil garlic mixture and place on a hot Panini press.

Close the Panini press and cook for 8–10 minutes or until golden brown.

In a mixing bowl, mix all topping ingredients.

Divide the topping mixture over toasted bread slices and serve.

Nutritional Data: 296 calories | 42.18g carbs | 8.39g fat | 15.79g protein | 570mg sodium

10-Spinach and Feta Phyllo Triangles

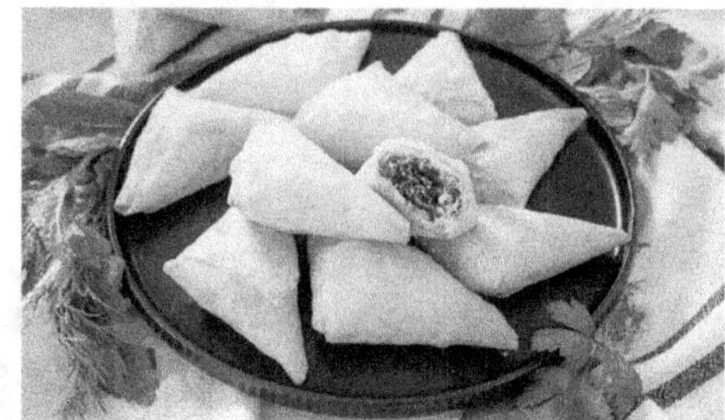

Preparation Time: 10 minutes
Cooking Time: 25 minutes
Serves: 20 triangles
Ingredients:

- 1 egg
- 5 phyllo pastry sheets
- 1 tbsp olive oil
- 1 spring onion, chopped
- 1 cup frozen spinach, cooked
- 1 cup feta cheese, crumbled
- Pepper
- Salt

Directions:

In a mixing bowl, mix together egg, crumbled cheese, spinach, spring onion, pepper, and salt until combined.

Place one phyllo sheet on the kitchen surface and brush lightly with oil. Hold it in half, then cut it into four strips.

Add a teaspoon of the spinach-cheese mixture right at the end of each strip, then fold it into a triangle. Repeat with the remaining phyllo sheets.

Preheat the oven to 350° F.

Place prepared triangles onto a parchment-lined baking sheet and bake in preheated oven for 25 minutes.

Serve and enjoy.

Nutritional Data: 50 calories | 3.45g carbs | 3.09g fat | 2.19g protein | 103mg sodium

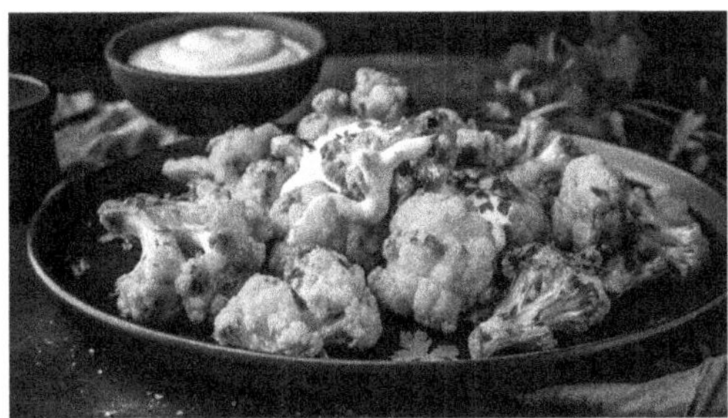

Preparation Time: 10 minutes
Cooking Time: 16 minutes
Serves: 4
Ingredients:

- 1 cauliflower head, cut into florets
- 1 tbsp butter, melted
- 1/2 cup buffalo sauce
- Pepper
- Salt

Directions:

Spray air fryer basket with cooking spray.

In a mixing bowl, mix buffalo sauce, butter, pepper, and salt.

Add cauliflower florets into the air fryer basket and cook at 400° F for 8 minutes.

Transfer cauliflower florets into the buffalo sauce mixture and toss well to coat.

Return cauliflower florets to the air fryer basket and cook for 8 minutes more.

Serve and enjoy.

Nutritional Data: 108 calories | 18.93g carbs | 3.31g fat | 1.82g protein | 411mg sodium

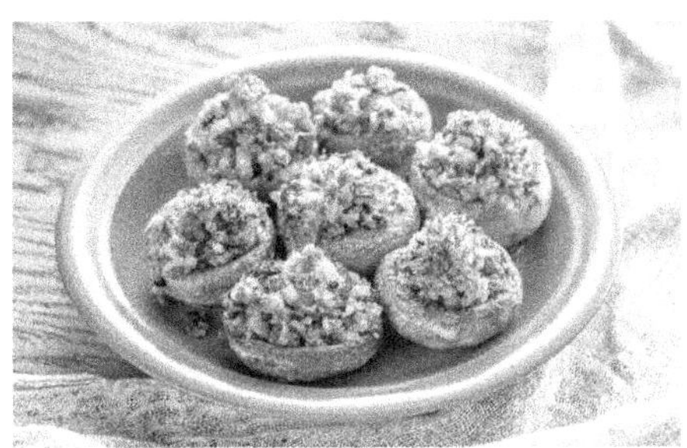

Preparation Time: 10 minutes
Cooking Time: 25 minutes
Serves: 16
Ingredients:

- 16 crimini mushrooms, stemmed
- ¼ cup olive oil
- ¼ cup pecans, chopped
- 2 tbsp parsley, chopped
- ¼ cup onion, minced
- 2 garlic cloves, minced
- ½ cup Romano cheese, shredded
- ½ cup cooked quinoa
- Pepper
- Salt

Directions:

Preheat the oven to 400° F.

In a medium bowl, mix together quinoa, pecans, 2 tablespoons of oil, parsley, onion, garlic, cheese, pepper, and salt.

Stuff the quinoa mixture into each mushroom cavity.

Arrange stuff mushrooms into the baking dish and drizzle with remaining olive oil.

Bake in preheated oven for 25 minutes.

Serve and enjoy.

Nutritional Data: 54 calories | 2.79g carbs | 4.63g fat | 0.95g protein | 2mg sodium

13-Avocado Cucumber Rolls

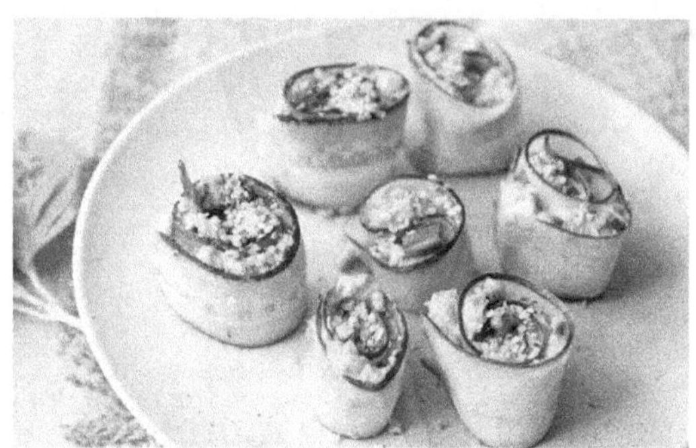

Preparation Time: 10 minutes
Cooking Time: 5 minutes
Serves: 2
Ingredients:

- 1 English cucumber, using a peeler slice the cucumber into thin strips
- 2 tbsp hemp seeds
- 2 tbsp mint, chopped
- 2 tbsp basil, chopped
- ½ lemon juice
- 1 avocado, mashed
- Pepper
- Salt

Directions:

In a bowl, mix together mashed avocado, lemon juice, pepper, and salt.

Place one strip of cucumber on the cutting board then spread some avocado mixture on the cucumber strip. Top with mint, basil, and hemp seeds and roll. Make the remaining cucumber strips roll.

Serve and enjoy.

Nutritional Data: 553 calories | 13.42g carbs | 36.7g fat | 44.63g protein | 96mg sodium

14-Zucchini Fritters

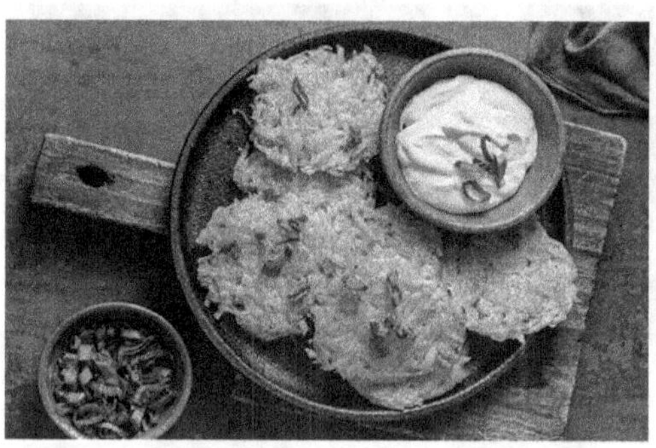

Preparation Time: 10 minutes
Cooking Time: 12 minutes
Serves: 4
Ingredients:

- 1 egg
- 3 medium zucchini, shredded & squeezed
- 1/4 tsp lemon pepper
- 1/2 tsp baking powder
- 1/4 cup parmesan cheese, grated
- 1/2 cup almond flour
- 2 green onions, chopped
- 1/2 tsp Italian seasoning
- 1/2 tsp paprika
- 1/2 tsp garlic powder
- Salt

Directions:

Preheat the oven to 350° F.

Line the baking sheet with parchment paper and set aside.

Add all ingredients into the bowl and mix until well combined.

Make patties from the mixture and place onto the prepared baking sheet.

Bake fritters in preheated oven for 10–12 minutes or until lightly golden and crispy.

Serve and enjoy.

Nutritional Data: 75 calories | 4.4g carbs | 4.47g fat | 4.74g protein | 170mg sodium

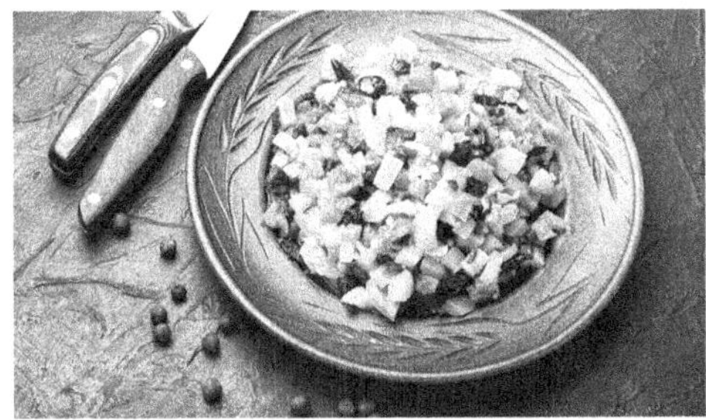

Preparation Time: 10 minutes
Cooking Time: 5 minutes
Serves: 4
Ingredients:

- 14-oz can low-sodium black beans, drained & rinsed
- 12-oz can corn, drained & rinsed
- ½ tsp cumin powder
- 4 tbsp olive oil
- 4 tbsp lime juice
- 1/3 cup cilantro, chopped
- 2 jalapenos, seeded & diced
- ½ onion, diced
- Pepper
- Salt

Directions:

In a mixing bowl, mix together black beans, corn, cumin powder, oil, lime juice, cilantro, jalapenos, and onion. Season salsa with pepper and salt.

Serve and enjoy.

Nutritional Data: 328 calories | 43.06g carbs | 14.53g fat | 10.83g protein | 226mg sodium

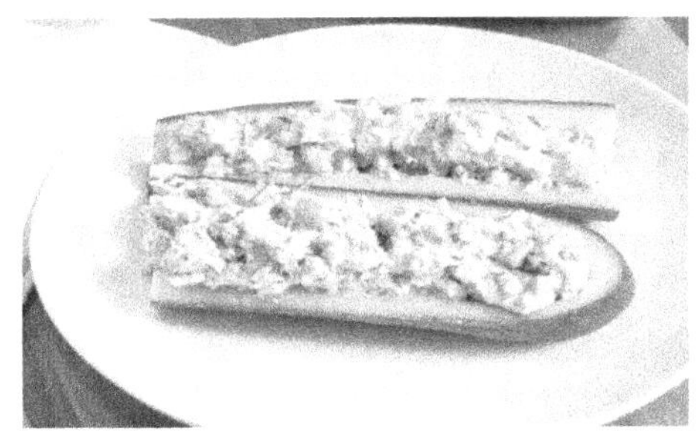

Preparation Time: 10 minutes
Cooking Time: 5 minutes
Serves: 4
Ingredients:

- 2 cucumbers, cut into slices & seeds scooped out with a spoon
- 3 oz wild albacore tuna
- ¼ tsp dill, chopped
- 1 tsp Dijon mustard
- 3 tbsp mayonnaise
- Pepper
- Salt

Directions:

In a medium bowl, mix tuna, mayonnaise, Dijon mustard, dill, pepper, and salt until combined.

Stuff a tablespoon of tuna mixture into each cucumber cup.

Serve immediately and enjoy.

Nutritional Data: 118 calories | 17.56g carbs | 3.89g fat | 4.12g protein | 103mg sodium

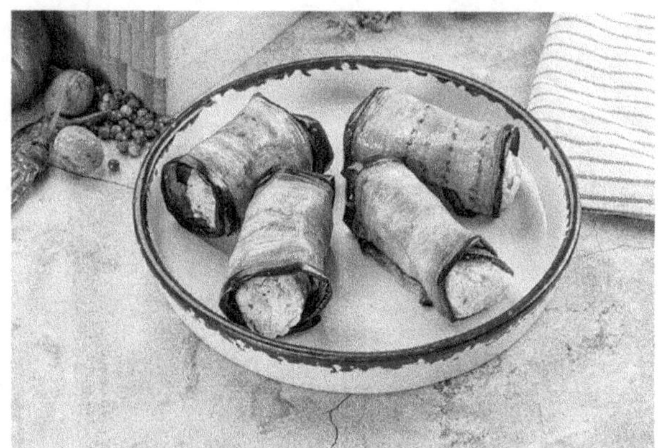

Preparation Time: 20 minutes
Cooking Time: 28 minutes
Serves: 6
Ingredients:

- 2 eggplants, sliced lengthwise into ¼-inch thick slices
- 2 cups marinara sauce
- 2 tbsp olive oil
- Salt
- For filling:
- 2 eggs, lightly beaten
- 1 cup parsley, chopped
- 2 tbsp basil pesto
- ¼ cup parmesan cheese, grated
- ½ cup mozzarella cheese, shredded
- 1 cup ricotta cheese

Directions:

Arrange eggplant slices on a plate and sprinkle with salt and set aside for 20 minutes.

After 20 minutes, rinse eggplant slices with water and pat dry with paper towels.

Preheat the oven to 375° F.

Arrange eggplant slices onto the baking sheet and brush with olive oil.

Bake in preheated oven for 8 minutes. Remove from oven and allow to cool completely.

In a medium bowl, mix eggs, parmesan cheese, mozzarella cheese, ricotta cheese,

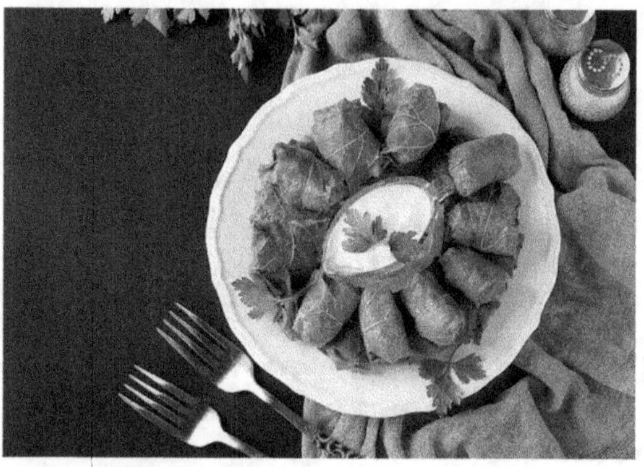

Preparation Time: 20 minutes
Cooking Time: 45 minutes
Serves: 8
Ingredients:

- 1 jar grape leaves
- ½ cup olive oil
- 1/3 cup parsley, chopped
- 2 tbsp pine nuts
- 1 tsp dried mint
- ½ tsp cinnamon
- 1 tsp tomato paste
- 1 cup short-grain rice
- 2 onions, chopped
- 2 tbsp vegetable oil
- Salt

Directions:

Heat vegetable oil in a pan over medium heat.

Add onion and sauté until softened. Add rice and cook for a few minutes.

Add tomato paste, parsley, pine nuts, mint, cinnamon, and salt, and stir well.

Add ½ cup hot water, stir well and cook for 5 minutes. Remove from heat.

Reserve five grape leaves to cover the bottom of the pot.

Place grape leaf on a clean kitchen surface. Add 1 tablespoon of rice mixture on the leaf and then roll the grape leaf parsley, and pesto until well combined.

Add ¾ cup marinara sauce onto the baking dish and spread well.

Add 2 tablespoons of the filling onto one end of each eggplant slice and spread evenly. Roll up eggplant slices tightly and place into the baking dish.

Add pesto, remaining marinara sauce, and some mozzarella cheese on top of the eggplant rolls and bake in preheated oven for 30 minutes.

Serve and enjoy.

Nutritional Data: 75 calories | 4.4g carbs | 4.47g fat | 4.74g protein | 170mg sodium

tightly.

Place reserved grape leaves in the bottom of a large pot then place stuffed grape leaves in the pot. Pour olive oil over stuffed grapes leaves.

Slowly pour hot water over the dolmas until it barely covers them.

Place one plate upside down on the stuffed grape leaves and cover with a lid.

Place pot on heat and cook over high heat until the water starts simmering. Turn heat to low and simmer for 45 minutes.

Serve and enjoy.

Nutritional Data: 363 calories | 43.58g carbs | 19.66g fat | 8.77g protein | 14mg sodium

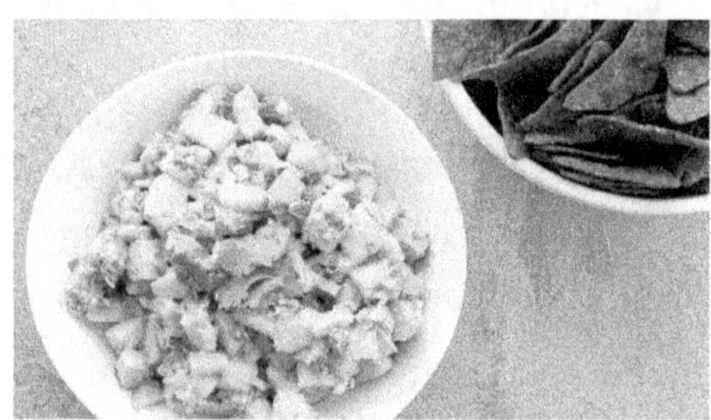

Preparation Time: 10 minutes
Cooking Time: 5 minutes
Serves: 4
Ingredients:

- 1 medium avocado, diced
- 1 ripe mango, peeled & diced
- ½ tbsp olive oil
- ¼ cup onion, chopped
- 2 tbsp lime juice
- ¼ cup cilantro, chopped
- 1 garlic, minced
- 1 tomato, diced
- Pepper
- Salt

Directions:

In a medium bowl, add avocado, mango and remaining ingredients and mix well.

Cover bowl and place in refrigerator for 30 minutes.

Serve and enjoy

Nutritional Data: 43 calories | 5.1g carbs | 2.68g fat | 0.72g protein | 2mg sodium

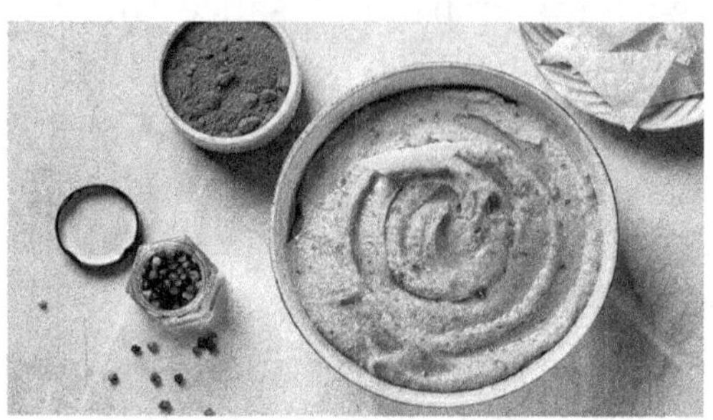

Preparation Time: 10 minutes
Cooking Time: 5 minutes
Serves: 8
Ingredients:

- 2 jars roasted red peppers
- 14-oz can chickpeas, rinsed & drained
- 2 tsp tahini
- 2 garlic cloves, minced
- 1 lemon, juiced
- 6 tbsp olive oil
- 1/4 tsp chili pepper flakes, crushed

Directions:

Add roasted red peppers, chickpeas, tahini, garlic, oil, and lemon juice into the food processor and process until smooth.

Garnish with crushed chili flakes and serve.

Nutritional Data: 203 calories | 18.61g carbs | 12.94g fat | 4.78g protein | 304mg sodium

21-Spinach-Artichoke-Stuffed Mushrooms

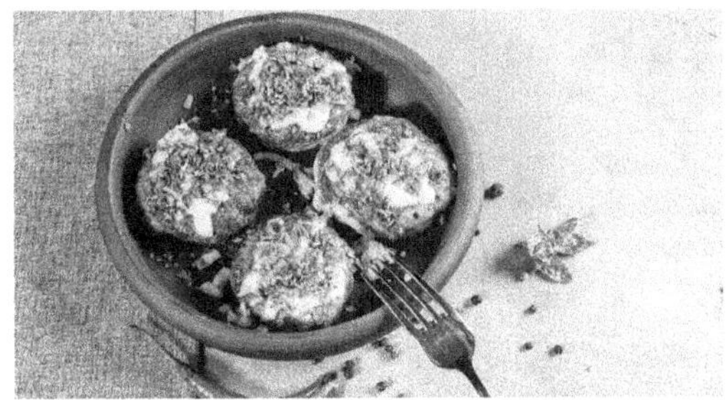

Preparation Time: 10 minutes
Cooking Time: 20 minutes
Serves: 30 mushrooms
Ingredients:

- 30 cremini mushrooms, stems removed
- ½ cup parmesan cheese, grated
- 10 oz frozen spinach, thawed & excess liquid squeezed out
- 14-oz can artichoke hearts, chopped
- 1 tsp garlic powder
- ½ cup sour cream
- ½ cup mayonnaise
- 4 oz cream cheese, softened
- Pepper
- Salt

Directions:

Preheat the oven to 400° F.

Lightly grease baking sheet with cooking spray and set aside.

In a mixing bowl, mix cream cheese, half parmesan cheese, spinach, artichoke hearts, garlic powder, sour cream, mayonnaise, pepper, and salt until combined.

Stuff spoonfuls of spinach artichoke mixture into the mushrooms.

Place mushrooms on the baking sheet and top with remaining parmesan cheese.

Bake in preheated oven for 18–20 minutes.

Serve and enjoy.

Nutritional Data: 50 calories | 3.35g carbs | 3.36g fat | 2.49g protein | 80mg sodium

22-Cucumber Dill Greek Yogurt Dip

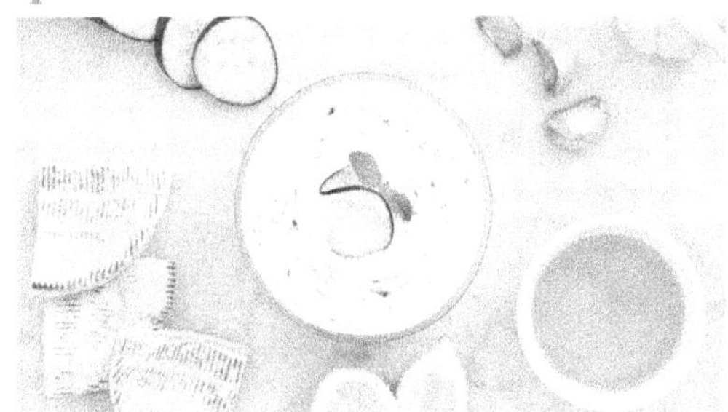

Preparation Time: 10 minutes
Cooking Time: 5 minutes
Serves: 4
Ingredients:

- 1 cup Greek yogurt
- 1 tbsp dill, chopped
- 1 cucumber, chopped
- ¼ tsp onion powder
- ¼ tsp garlic powder
- 1 tbsp lemon juice
- Pepper
- Salt

Directions:

In a medium bowl, mix together yogurt, dill, cucumber, onion powder, garlic powder, lemon juice, pepper, and salt until combined.

Cover and place in refrigerator for 30 minutes.

Serve and enjoy.

Nutritional Data: 127 calories | 5g carbs | 2.11g fat | 2.71g protein | 30mg sodium

23-Tomato Basil Mozzarella Skewers

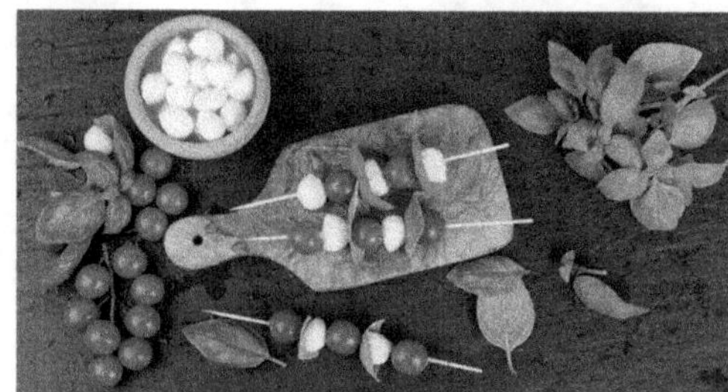

Preparation Time: 10 minutes
Cooking Time: 5 minutes
Serves: 4
Ingredients:

- 2 cups grape tomatoes
- ½ cup fresh basil leaves
- ¼ cup olive oil
- 1 cup mozzarella balls
- Salt

Directions:

In a mixing bowl, mix olive oil, tomatoes, mozzarella balls, and salt.

Thread tomatoes, basil leaves, and mozzarella balls alternatively onto wooden skewers.

Serve and enjoy.

Nutritional Data: 132 calories | 17g carbs | 13g fat | 0.91g protein | 15mg sodium

24-Cucumber Hummus Bites

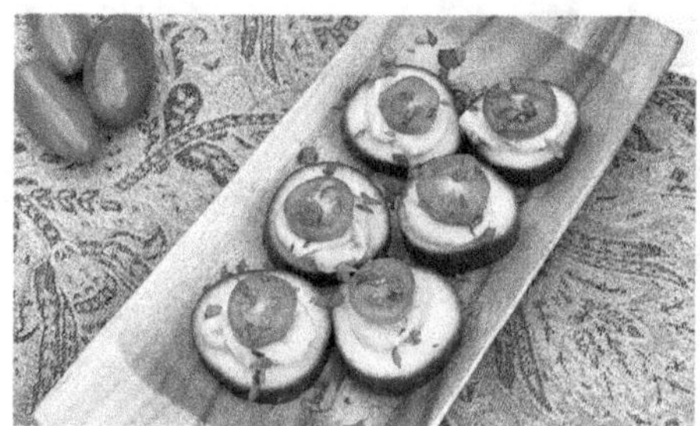

Preparation Time: 10 minutes
Cooking Time: 5 minutes
Serves: 4
Ingredients:

- 2 cups grape tomatoes
- ½ cup fresh basil leaves
- ¼ cup olive oil
- 1 cup mozzarella balls
- Salt

Directions:

Arrange cucumber slices on a serving platter and top with 1 tablespoon of hummus.

Top each slice with cherry tomatoes.

Serve immediately and enjoy.

Nutritional Data: 387 calories | 39g carbs | 24g fat | 7.2g protein | 20mg sodium

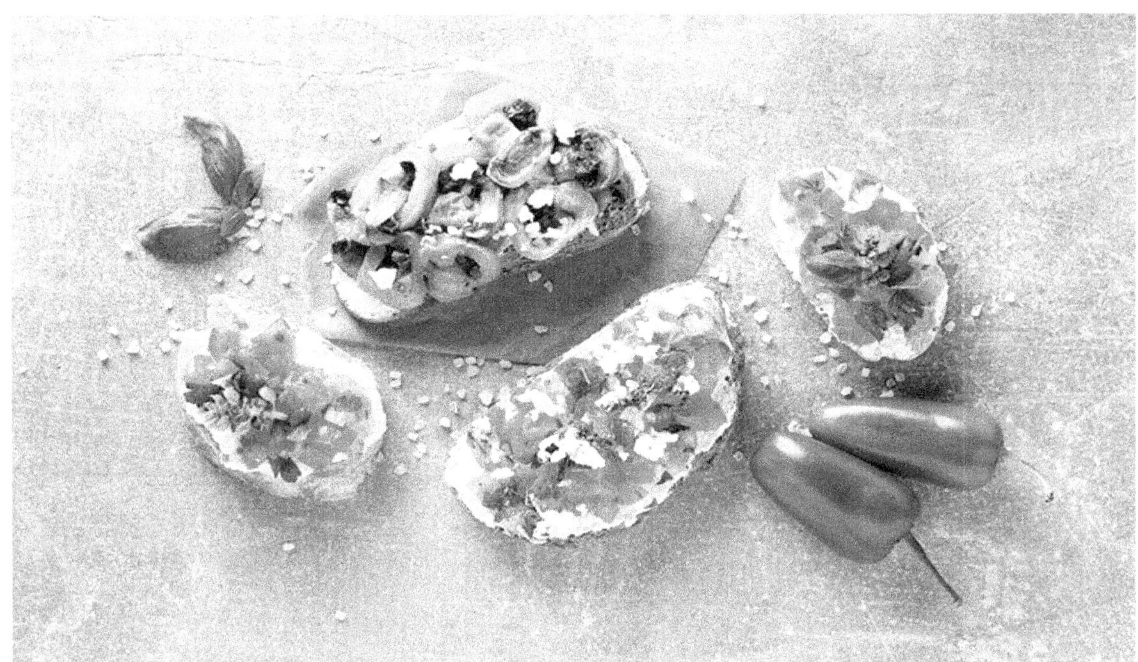

Preparation Time: 10 minutes
Cooking Time: 50 minutes
Serves: 4
Ingredients:
- 8 oz whole-wheat baguette bread, cut into 1-inch slices
- 2 tbsp garlic, minced
- 2 tbsp olive oil
- 2 cups bell peppers, cut into 1-inch pieces
- 1 cup tomatoes, cut into 1-inch pieces
- 1 cup yellow squash, cut into 1-inch pieces
- 1 cup zucchini, cut into 1-inch pieces
- 1 cup eggplant, cut into 1-inch pieces
- 3 tbsp vegetable oil
- 0.84 oz vegetable bruschetta seasoning

Directions:

Preheat the oven to 425° F.

In a mixing bowl, add vegetables, seasoning, and vegetable oil and toss to coat well.

Spread vegetables on foil-lined baking sheet and roast in preheated oven for 35–40 minutes. Stir vegetables halfway through.

Preheat the Panini press.

In a small bowl, mix oil and garlic.

Brush bread slices with oil-garlic mixture and place on hot Panini press. In batches.

Close the Panini press and cook for 8–10 minutes or until golden brown.

Divide the roasted vegetable over toasted bread slices and serve.

Nutritional Data: 183 calories | 23g carbs | 7.97g fat | 4.7g protein | 144mg sodium

Chapter 4 — Snack Recipes

1-Greek Yogurt with Berries

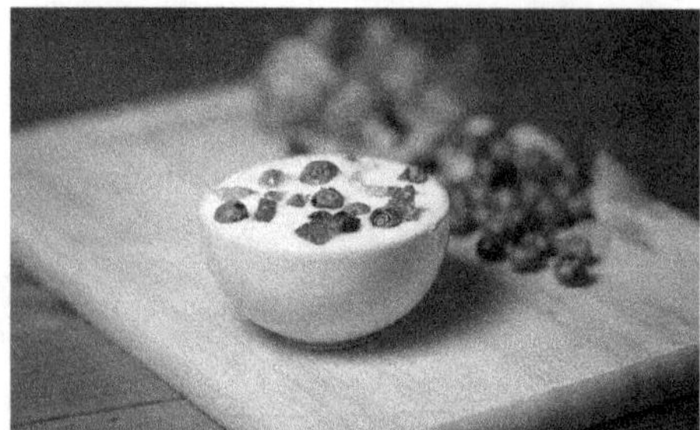

Preparation Time: 10 minutes
Cooking Time: 5 minutes
Serves: 1
Ingredients:

- 3/4 cup Greek yogurt
- 1 tbsp honey
- 1/4 cup fresh blueberries
- 1/4 cup fresh raspberries
- 1/4 cup fresh blackberries
- 3/4 cup fresh strawberries, chopped

Directions:

Add yogurt to a serving bowl then top with berries.

Drizzle with honey and serve.

Nutritional Data: 390 calories | 76.65g carbs | 1.48g fat | 22.95g protein | 80mg sodium

2-Apple Slices with Almond Butter

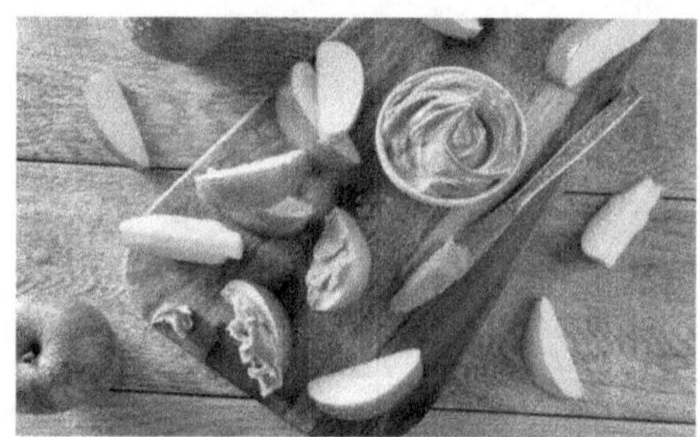

Preparation Time: 5 minutes
Cooking Time: 5 minutes
Serves: 2
Ingredients:

- 2 apples, cored & sliced
- ½ tsp vanilla
- ¼ tsp cinnamon
- 2 tbsp unsweetened almond milk
- ¼ cup almond butter

Directions:

In a small bowl, mix almond butter, cinnamon, vanilla, and almond milk until smooth.

Serve with sliced apples.

Nutritional Data: 298 calories | 32.84g carbs | 17.85g fat | 7.13g protein | 84mg sodium

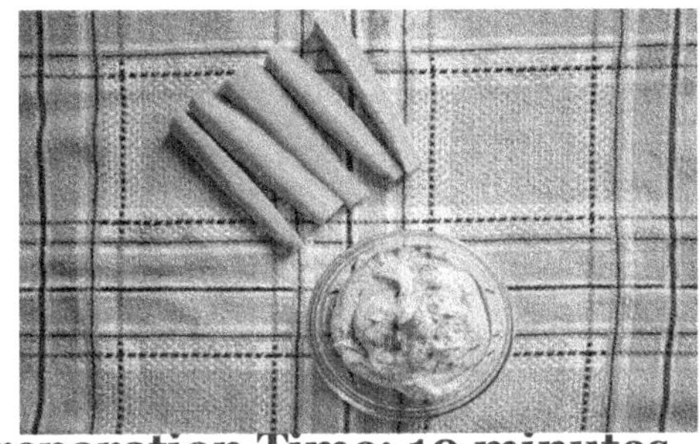

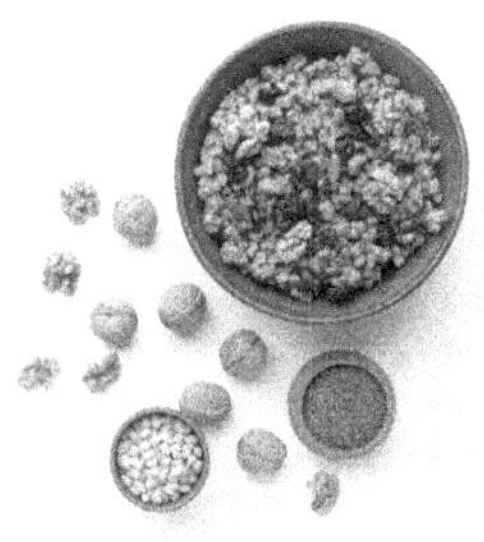

3-Carrot Sticks with Hummus

Preparation Time: 10 minutes
Cooking Time: 5 minutes
Serves: 4
Ingredients:

- 10-oz can chickpeas, drained & rinsed
- 1 garlic clove
- 4 tbsp olive oil
- ¼ tsp ground cumin
- ½ lemon, juiced
- Salt
- 2 medium carrots, peeled & cut into small spears

Directions:

Add chickpeas, garlic, olive oil, cumin, lemon juice, and salt into the blender and blend until smooth.

Transfer hummus to a serving bowl and serve with carrot sticks.

Nutritional Data: 233 calories | 19.85g carbs | 15.37g fat | 5.36g protein | 172mg sodium

4-Trail Mix

Preparation Time: 5 minutes
Cooking Time: 5 minutes
Serves: 8
Ingredients:

- 6 dates, pitted & chopped
- 4 tbsp raisins
- 4 tbsp dried cranberries
- 1/3 cup pumpkin seeds
- 1/3 cup dried apricots
- ½ cup almonds
- ½ cup walnuts
- Pinch of salt

Directions:

In a mixing bowl, mix dates, raisins, cranberries, pumpkin seeds, apricots, almonds, and walnuts.

Sprinkle with a pinch of salt.

Store in a container with a lid.

Nutritional Data: 94 calories | 10.05g carbs | 5.74g fat | 2.55g protein | 13mg sodium

5-Whole Grain Crackers with Cottage Cheese

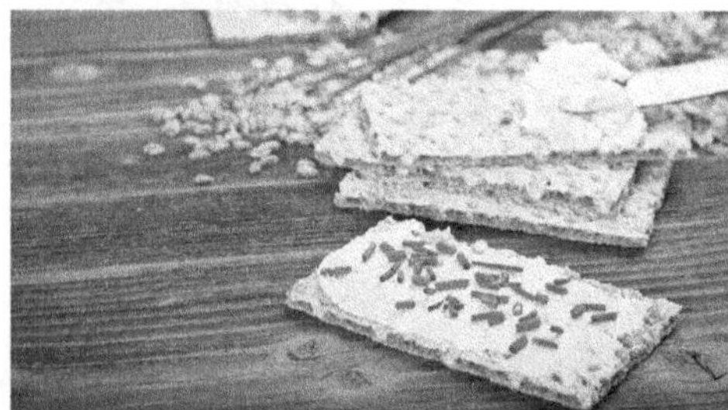

Preparation Time: 10 minutes
Cooking Time: 25 minutes
Serves: 4
Ingredients:

- 1 ½ cups rolled oats
- ½ cup water
- 6 tbsp olive oil
- 2 tbsp ground flax seeds
- ½ cup wheat germ
- 1 cup whole wheat flour
- ¼ tsp salt
- For cottage cheese:
- 1 cup cottage cheese
- 1 tsp lemon juice
- 1 tsp garlic, minced
- 1/8 tsp pepper

Directions:

In a bowl, mix cottage cheese, lemon juice, garlic, and pepper until well combined. Set aside.

Add oats, flax seeds, wheat germ, whole wheat flour, and salt into the food processor. Slowly add oil and water and process until well combined.

Divide dough between two cookie sheets and roll until thin.

Cut into square pieces and place on a parchment-lined baking sheet.

Bake in preheated oven at 350° F for 20 minutes.

Serve crackers with cottage cheese.

Nutritional Data: 516 calories | 56.58g carbs | 30.74g fat | 20.64g protein | 347mg sodium

6-Deviled Eggs

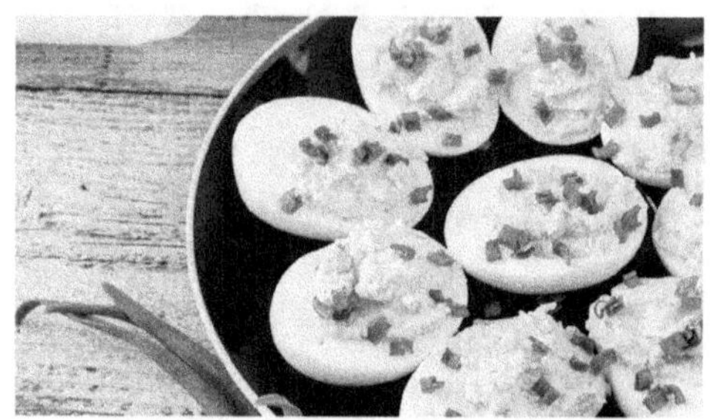

Preparation Time: 10 minutes
Cooking Time: 10 minutes
Serves: 12
Ingredients:

- 6 hard-boiled eggs, peeled
- 2 tbsp onion, diced
- 2 tbsp mayonnaise
- 1 avocado, diced
- 1 tsp fresh cilantro, chopped
- 1/4 fresh lime juice
- Pepper
- Salt

Directions:

Cut eggs in half lengthwise.

Add egg yolks to the mixing bowl and place egg whites onto a serving plate.

Add avocado into a mixing bowl and mash with egg yolk.

Add onion, mayonnaise, cilantro, lime juice, pepper, and salt and mix well.

Spoon the avocado mixture evenly into the egg white halves.

Serve and enjoy.

Nutritional Data: 76 calories | 2.37g carbs | 5.91g fat | 3.73g protein | 52mg sodium

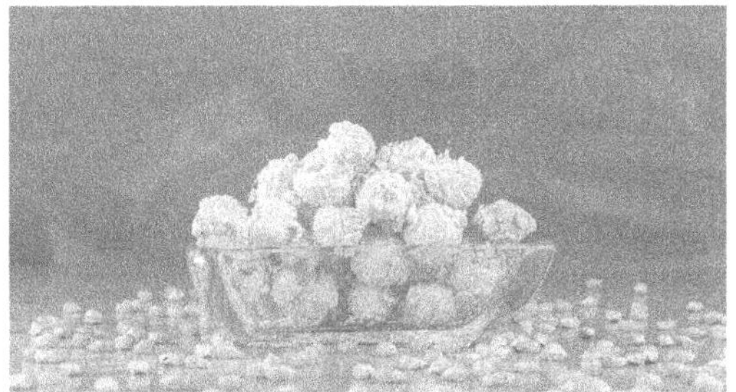

Preparation Time: 5 minutes
Cooking Time: 4 minutes
Serves: 8
Ingredients:

- ½ cup popcorn kernels
- ½ tsp olive oil
- Salt

Directions:

In a small bowl, mix popcorn kernels with oil.

Add popcorn kernels in a paper bag and fold over the top.

Place in oven and microwave for 2–4 minutes.

Remove the bag from the oven and pour the popcorn into a bowl.

Sprinkle with salt and serve.

Nutritional Data: 36 calories | 5.69g carbs | 1.02g fat | 0.98g protein | 38mg sodium

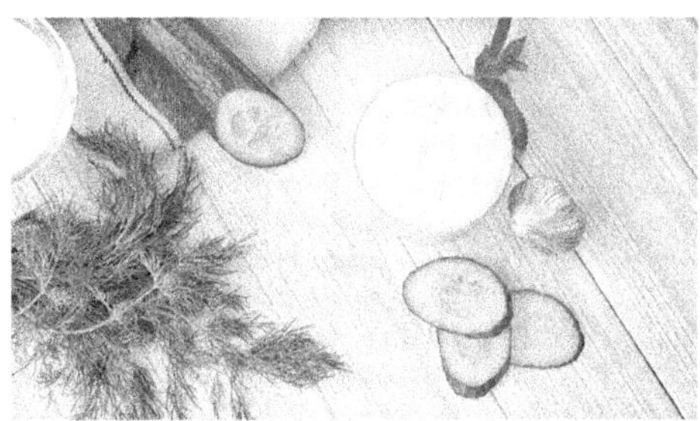

Preparation Time: 10 minutes
Cooking Time: 10 minutes
Serves: 6
Ingredients:

- 1 English cucumber, peeled & cut into thick slices
- 1 tbsp olive oil
- 2 tbsp dill, chopped
- 1 garlic, chopped
- ¼ lemon, juiced
- 6 oz Greek yogurt
- Salt

Directions:

Arrange cucumber slices on a serving platter.

In a bowl, mix yogurt, oil, dill, garlic, lemon juice, and salt until well combined.

Dollop a teaspoon of yogurt mixture on top of each cucumber slice.

Serve immediately and enjoy.

Nutritional Data: 44 calories | 2.4g carbs | 2.69g fat | 3.25g protein | 11mg sodium

9-Rice Cakes with Peanut Butter

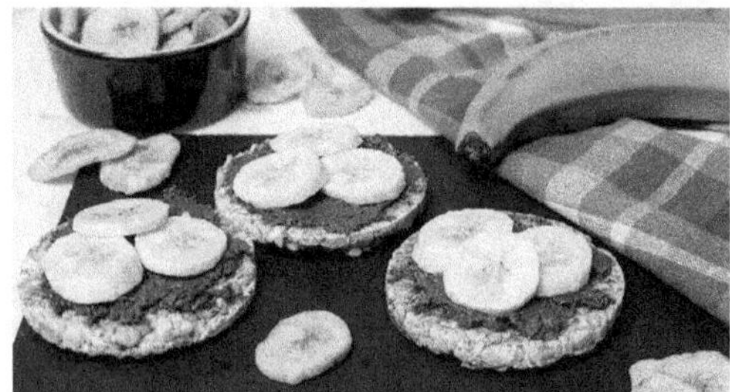

Preparation Time: 5 minutes
Cooking Time: 10 minutes
Serves: 4
Ingredients:

- 4 brown rice cakes, lightly salted
- 4 tbsp peanut butter
- 2 bananas, cut into slices

Directions:

- Spread one tablespoon of peanut butter on each rice cake then top each rice cake with ½ banana slices.
- Serve and enjoy.

Nutritional Data: 81 calories | 11.3g carbs | 3.14g fat | 1.87g protein | 270mg sodium

10-Cherry Tomatoes with Mozzarella

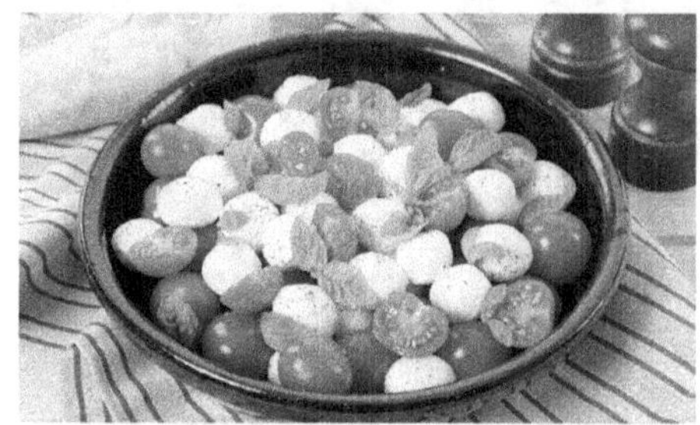

Preparation Time: 10 minutes
Cooking Time: 5 minutes
Serves: 6
Ingredients:

- 2 cups mozzarella balls, cut in half
- 4 cups cherry tomatoes, cut in half
- ¼ tsp garlic powder
- ¼ tsp dried oregano
- 1 ½ tbsp red wine vinegar
- ¼ cup olive oil
- 2 tbsp basil, chopped
- 2 tbsp parsley, chopped
- 4 tbsp onion, minced
- Pepper
- Salt

Directions:

Add mozzarella balls, cherry tomatoes, and remaining ingredients into the mixing bowl and mix until well coated.

Serve and enjoy.

Nutritional Data: 136 calories | 9.41g carbs | 10.13g fat | 2.39g protein | 79mg sodium

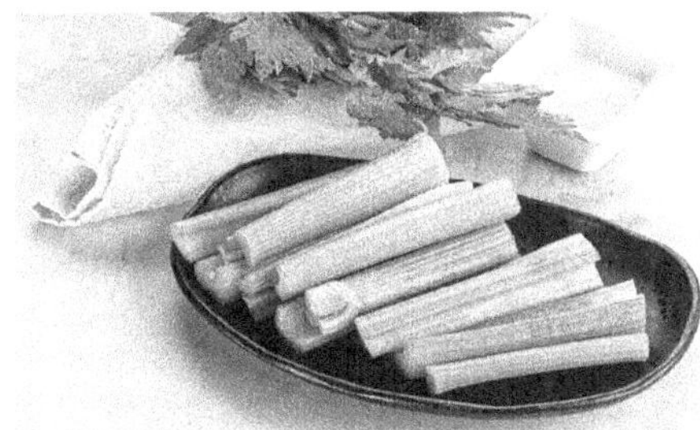

Preparation Time: 5 minutes
Cooking Time: 5 minutes
Serves: 1
Ingredients:

- 4 brown rice cakes, lightly salted
- 4 tbsp peanut butter
- 2 bananas, cut into slices

Directions:

Cut celery stalks into 3-inch pieces.

Spread almond butter to the center of celery stalks.

Serve and enjoy.

Nutritional Data: 106 calories | 4.53g carbs | 8.97g fat | 3.71g protein | 77mg sodium

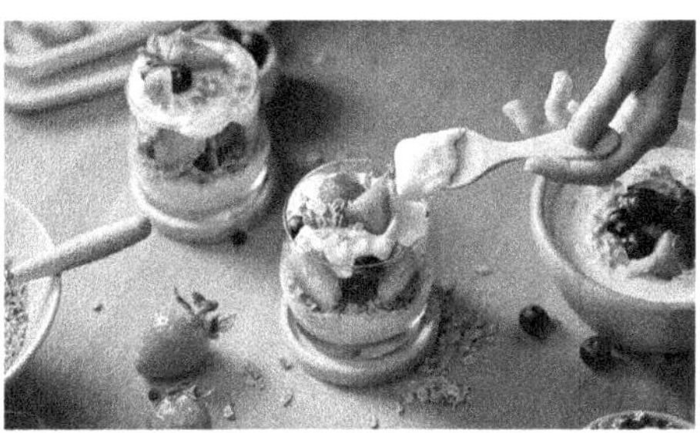

Preparation Time: 10 minutes
Cooking Time: 5 minutes
Serves: 4
Ingredients:

- 32 oz Greek yogurt
- ½ cup walnuts, chopped
- ½ cup pecans, chopped
- 1 cup granola
- 2 cups raspberries
- 2 cups blueberries
- 2 cups strawberries, sliced

Directions:

Add ½ cup yogurt to the bottom of four serving cups.

Top with ¼ cup raspberries, blueberries, and strawberries in each cup.

Add granola, walnuts, and pecans on top of berries in each cup.

Cover and place in refrigerator until serving.

Serve and enjoy.

Nutritional Data: 684 calories | 89.8g carbs | 25.68g fat | 30.79g protein | 143mg sodium

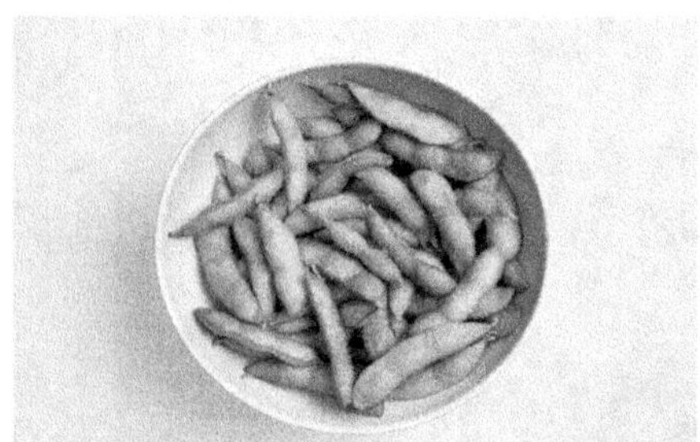

Preparation Time: 5 minutes
Cooking Time: 10 minutes
Serves: 4
Ingredients:

- 10 oz frozen edamame, shelled
- 1/4 tsp paprika
- 2 tbsp olive oil
- Pepper
- Salt

Directions:

In a bowl, toss edamame with paprika, oil, pepper, and salt.

Add edamame into the air fryer basket and cook at 400° F for 10 minutes. Stir halfway through.

Serve and enjoy.

Nutritional Data: 151 calories | 8.19g carbs | 10.48g fat | 7.96g protein | 5mg sodium

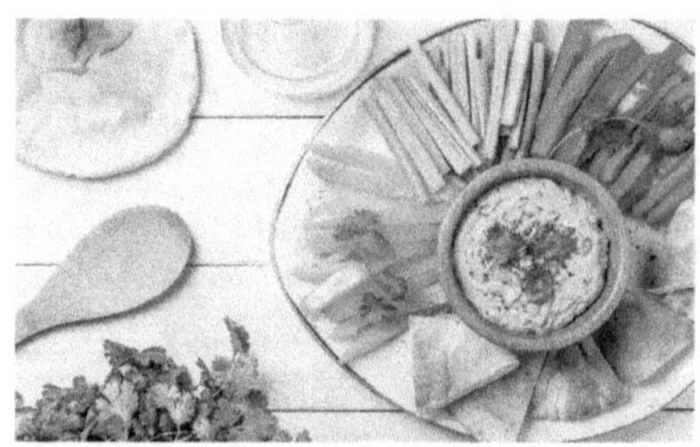

Preparation Time: 10 minutes
Cooking Time: 25 minutes
Serves: 4
Ingredients:

- 1 cup dry chickpeas, soaked overnight & drained
- 1/2 cup olive oil
- 1 tsp ground cumin
- 2 green chilies
- 1/2 cup fresh parsley
- 1 tbsp tahini
- 4 garlic cloves
- Pepper
- Salt
- 2 yellow bell pepper, seeds removed & cut into strips
- 2 red bell pepper, seeds removed & cut into strips

Directions:

Add chickpeas into the instant pot and cover with water.

Cover the pot with a lid and cook on high pressure for 25 minutes.

Allow to release pressure naturally. Remove lid.

Drain the chickpeas and transfer them into the food processor.

Add remaining ingredients and process until smooth.

Serve with bell pepper strips.

Nutritional Data: 754 calories | 26.44g carbs | 69.03g fat | 16.3g protein | 119mg sodium

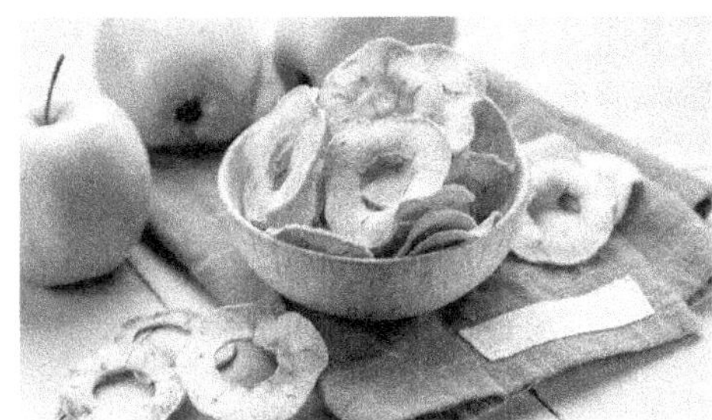

Preparation Time: 5 minutes
Cooking Time: 2 hours
Serves: 4
Ingredients:

- 2 apples, cored & cut into thin slices
- 1 tsp cinnamon

Directions:

Preheat the oven to 240° F.

Arrange apple slices on a baking sheet and sprinkle with cinnamon.

Bake in preheated oven for 2 hours. Remove from oven and allow to cool completely.

Serve and enjoy.

Nutritional Data: 49 calories | 13.09g carbs | 0.16g fat | 0.26g protein | 1mg sodium

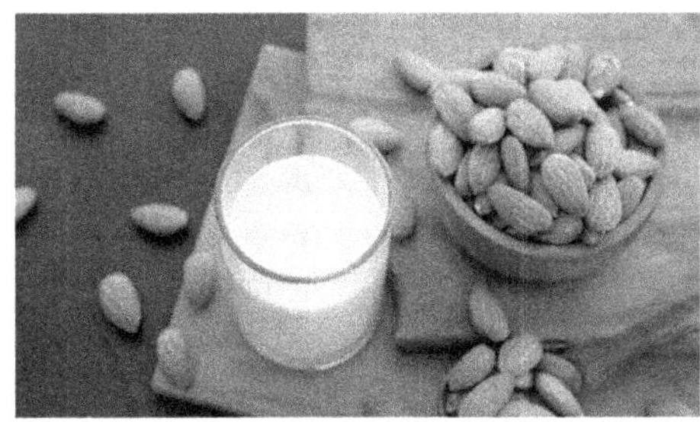

Preparation Time: 10 minutes
Cooking Time: 20 minutes
Serves: 12
Ingredients:

- 2 1/2 cups almonds
- 1/4 teaspoon cumin powder
- 1/4 teaspoon chili powder
- 1 tablespoon olive oil
- 2 1/2 tablespoons maple syrup
- 1/8 teaspoon cayenne
- 1 tablespoon fresh rosemary, chopped
- 1/4 teaspoon ground coriander
- Salt

Directions:

Preheat the oven to 325° F.

In a bowl, mix oil, coriander, cumin, chili powder, rosemary, cayenne, maple syrup, and salt.

Add almonds and toss until well coated.

Spread almonds on a baking sheet and roast in preheated oven for 20 minutes. Stir halfway through.

Serve and enjoy.

Nutritional Data: 23 calories | 2.93g carbs | 1.28g fat | 0.08g protein | 2mg sodium

17-Greek Yogurt Dip with Veggie Sticks

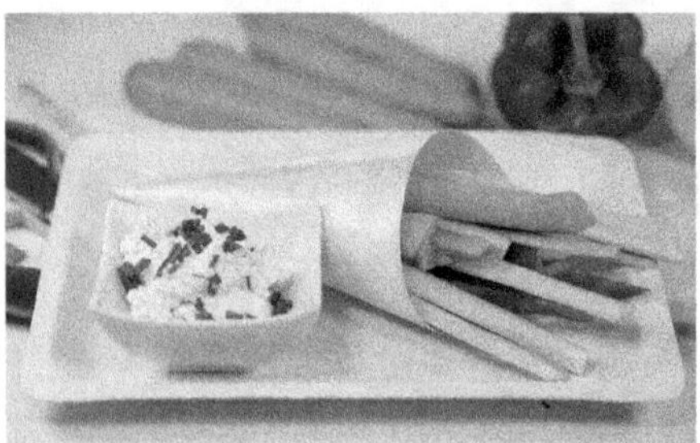

Preparation Time: 10 minutes
Cooking Time: 5 minutes
Serves: 4
Ingredients:

- 1 ½ cups Greek yogurt
- 2 tbsp lemon juice
- ½ tsp onion powder
- ½ tsp garlic powder
- 3 tbsp dill, chopped
- 2 tbsp mayonnaise
- Pepper
- Salt
- 2 carrots, peeled & cut into sticks
- 2 celery stalks, cut into 3-inch pieces
- 2 bell peppers, seeds removed & cut into strips

Directions:

In a bowl, mix together yogurt, lemon juice, onion powder, garlic powder, dill, mayonnaise, pepper, and salt until combined.

Serve dip with veggie sticks.

Nutritional Data: 174 calories | 12.74g carbs | 10.54g fat | 10.54g protein | 111mg sodium

18-Whole Grain Toast with Avocado

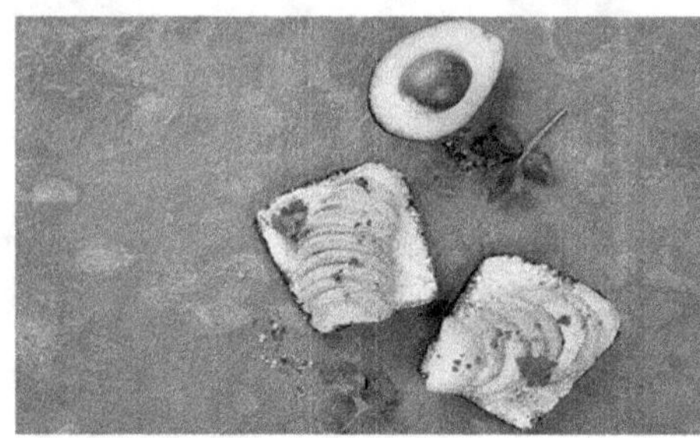

Preparation Time: 10 minutes
Cooking Time: 5 minutes
Serves: 4
Ingredients:

- 2 avocados, flesh scooped out
- 4 whole grain bread slices
- 1/4 cup kalamata olives, pitted
- 1/4 cup feta cheese, crumbled
- 1/4 cup fresh dill, chopped
- Pepper
- Salt

Directions:

Toast bread slices in a pan over high heat for 1–2 minutes on each side.

Add avocado flesh into the bowl and mash using a fork.

Add olives, crumbled cheese, dill, pepper, and salt, and mix until well combined.

Spread avocado mixture on top of toasted bread slices and serve.

Nutritional Data: 309 calories | 28.35g carbs | 19.39g fat | 9.13g protein | 312mg sodium

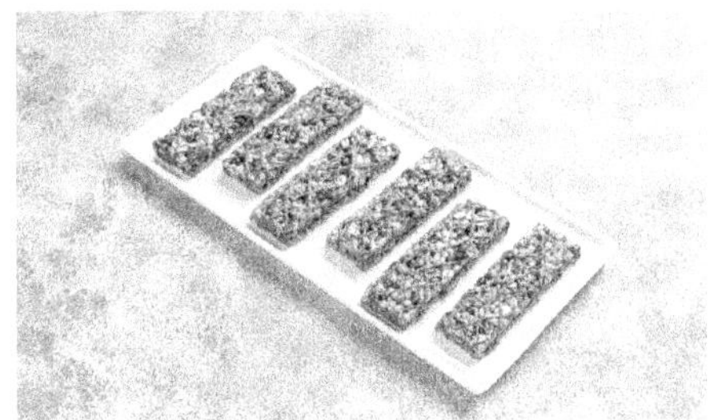

Preparation Time: 10 minutes
Cooking Time: 15 minutes
Serves: 12
Ingredients:

- 2 cups quick oats
- ½ cup unsweetened chocolate chips
- ¼ cup honey
- 1 cup creamy almond butter
- ½ tsp cinnamon
- ½ cup almonds, sliced
- Salt

Directions:

Line 8x8-inch baking dish with parchment paper and set aside.

In a medium bowl, mix together oats, chocolate chips, honey, almond, almond butter, cinnamon, and salt until well combined.

Add the oat mixture onto the prepared baking dish and spread evenly. Place in the freezer for 50 minutes or until firm.

Cut into pieces and serve.

Nutritional Data: 243 calories | 24.65g carbs | 14.39g fat | 6.61g protein | 83mg sodium

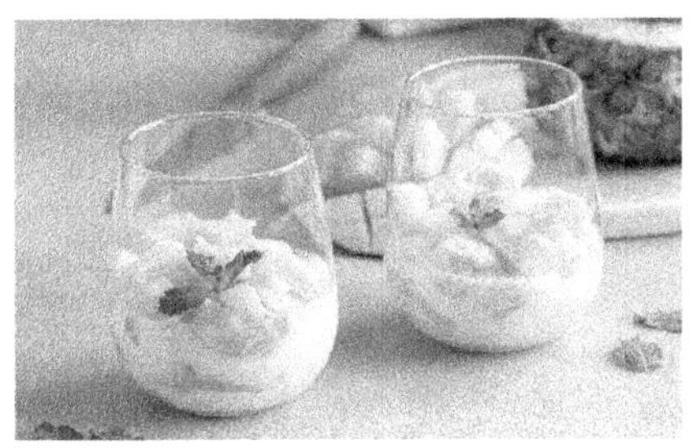

Preparation Time: 5 minutes
Cooking Time: 10 minutes
Serves: 4
Ingredients:

- 10 oz pineapple chunks
- 16 oz cottage cheese
- Fresh mint leaves

Directions:

Divide cottage cheese into four serving cups.

Add pineapple chunks on top of cottage cheese.

Garnish with fresh mint leaves and serve.

Nutritional Data: 172 calories | 19.57g carbs | 4.95g fat | 12.89g protein | 414mg sodium

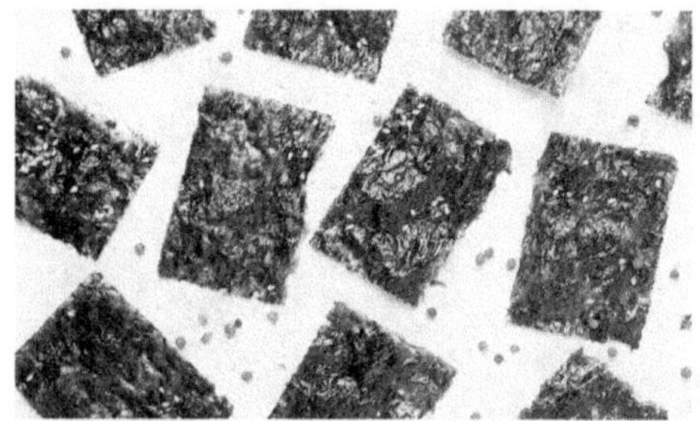

Preparation Time: 10 minutes
Cooking Time: 6 minutes
Serves: 4
Ingredients:
- 2 nori sheets
- 2 tbsp olive oil
- Salt

Directions:

Preheat the oven to 340° F.

Cut each nori sheet into six small pieces.

Brush the shiny side of each nori piece with oil and sprinkle with salt.

Place all nori pieces onto a baking sheet and bake in preheated oven for 6 minutes.

Serve and enjoy.

Nutritional Data: 60 calories | 0g carbs | 6.75g fat | 0g protein | 0mg sodium

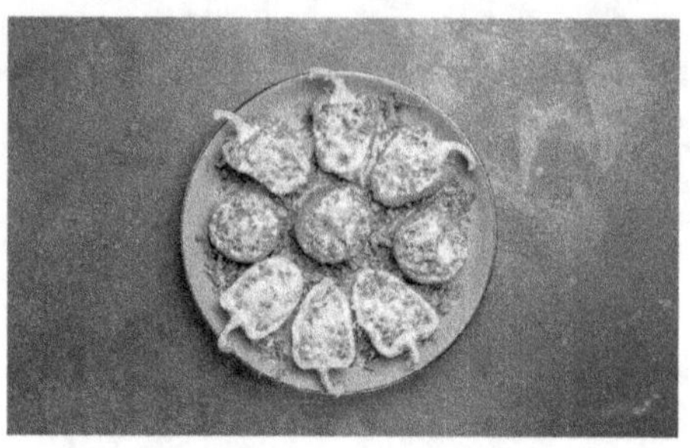

Preparation Time: 10 minutes
Cooking Time: 20 minutes
Serves: 6
Ingredients:
- 12 mini peppers, cut in half & seeds removed
- 2 tsp lemon juice
- 1 lemon, zested
- 1 green onion, chopped
- 1 tsp olive oil
- 24 olives, pitted & chopped
- 4 oz goat cheese

Directions:

Preheat the oven to 350° F.

In a bowl, mix together goat cheese, olives, oil, green onion, lemon zest, and lemon juice until combined.

Stuff the cheese mixture into each pepper half.

Arrange stuff peppers on the baking sheet and bake in preheated oven for 20 minutes.

Serve and enjoy.

Nutritional Data: 164 calories | 3.66g carbs | 13.91g fat | 7.52g protein | 250mg sodium

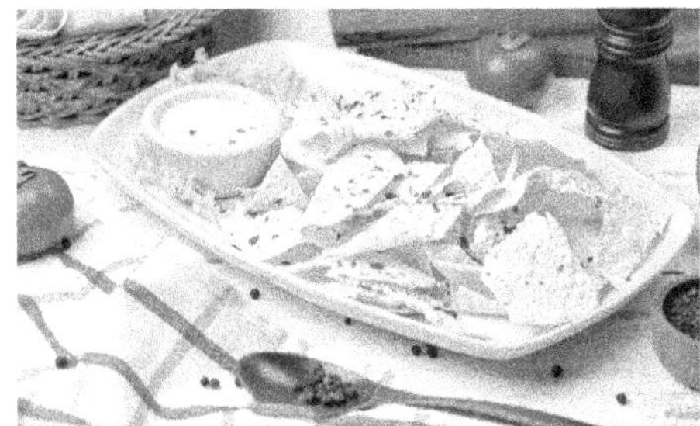

Preparation Time: 10 minutes
Cooking Time: 40 minutes
Serves: 6
Ingredients:

- For dip:
- 2 cups Greek yogurt
- 1 tsp onion powder
- 1 ½ tsp garlic powder
- 4 tsp apple cider vinegar
- 1 tbsp dill, minced
- 3 tbsp parsley, minced
- Pepper
- Salt
- For pita chips:
- 4 round whole grain pita bread
- 1 tbsp olive oil
- Pepper
- Salt

Directions:

For dip: In a bowl, mix yogurt, onion powder, garlic powder, vinegar, dill, parsley, pepper, and salt until combined. Set aside.

For pita chips: Cut pita bread into triangles and spread onto a baking sheet. Brush with oil and season with pepper and salt.

Bake in the oven for 8–10 minutes at 400° F or until crispy. Remove from oven and let it cool.

Serve baked pita bread chips with yogurt dip.

Nutritional Data: 97 calories | 9.43g carbs | 3.08g fat | 8.61g protein | 59mg sodium

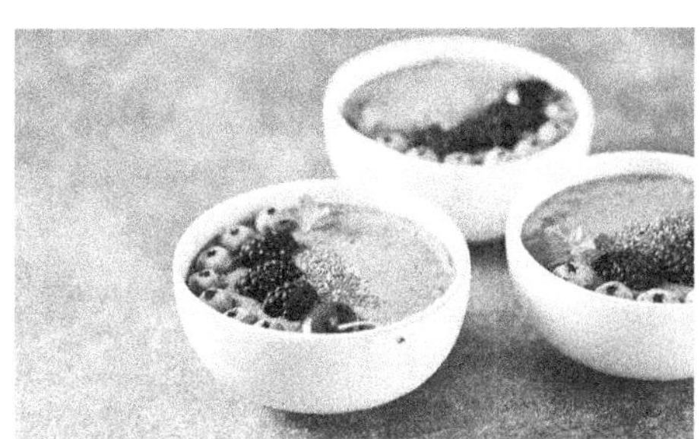

Preparation Time: 5 minutes
Cooking Time: 5 minutes
Serves: 2
Ingredients:

- ¼ cup chia seeds
- 2 tbsp honey
- ½ tsp vanilla
- 1 cup unsweetened almond milk
- 1 cup raspberries

Directions:

Add raspberries, almond milk, vanilla, and honey into the blender and blend until smooth.

Transfer blended mixture into the bowl.

Add chia seeds and stir well. Cover and place in refrigerator for 3 hours.

Stir well and serve.

Nutritional Data: 348 calories | 67.65g carbs | 8.26g fat | 5.44g protein | 93mg sodium

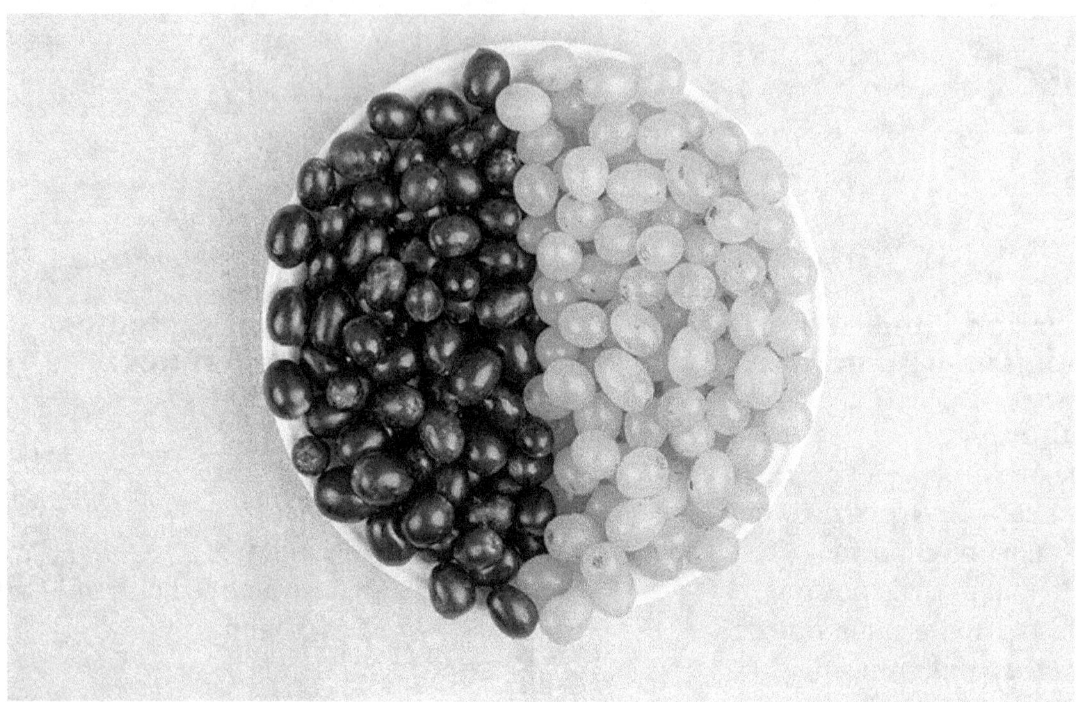

Preparation Time: 5 minutes
Cooking Time: 5 minutes
Serves: 2
Ingredients:

- 1 ½ cups white grapes
- 1 ½ cups red grapes

Directions:

Add grapes in a colander and rinse them for 40 seconds to remove pesticides and bacteria.

Gently pull the grapes from the stem.

Add grapes into a zip-lock bag and place in the freezer overnight.

Serve and enjoy.

Nutritional Data: 156 calories | 41g carbs | 0.36g fat | 1.63g protein | 5mg sodium

Chapter 5 — Lunch Recipes

1-Mediterranean Chickpea Salad

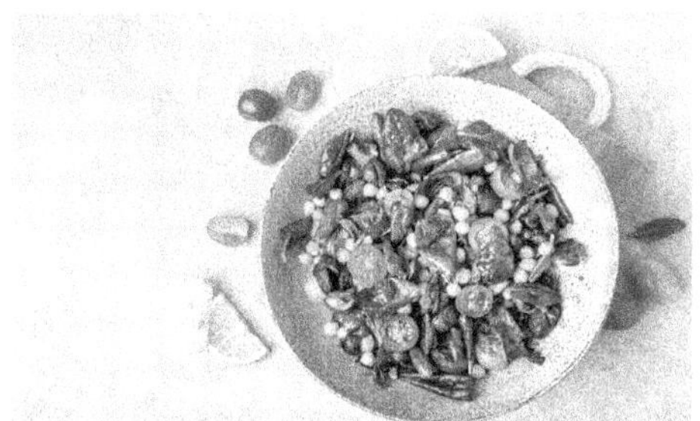

Preparation Time: 10 minutes
Cooking Time: 5 minutes
Serves: 6
Ingredients:

- 15-oz can chickpeas, drained & rinsed
- 1 tbsp capers, drained & chopped
- 1 tbsp rosemary, chopped
- 1/4 cup vinegar
- 1/3 cup fresh basil, chopped
- 1/3 cup olive oil
- 1/2 cup olives, chopped
- 1/2 cup feta cheese, crumbled
- 1/2 cup onion, chopped
- 2 cups zucchini, diced
- 1/8 tsp red pepper flakes
- 1/2 tsp dried oregano
- 1 garlic clove, minced
- 3/4 cup bell pepper, chopped
- 1 cup cherry tomatoes, halved
- Pepper
- Salt

Directions:

Add all ingredients into a large bowl and mix everything well.

Serve and enjoy.

Nutritional Data: 264 calories | 20.47g carbs | 17.59g fat | 7.49g protein | 383mg sodium

2-Quinoa and Black Bean-Stuffed Bell Peppers

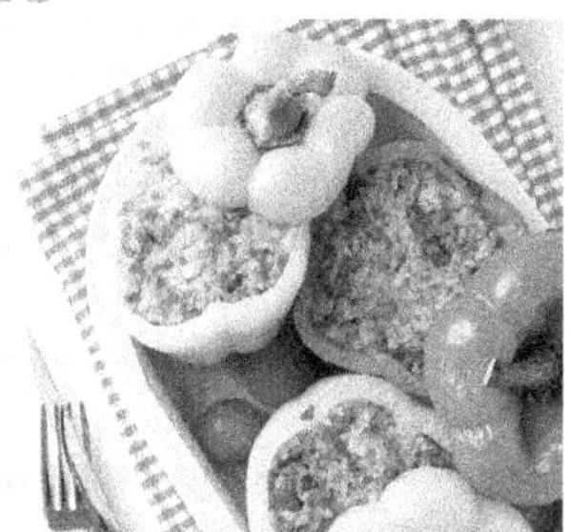

Preparation Time: 10 minutes
Cooking Time: 25 minutes
Serves: 6
Ingredients:

- 1 cup quinoa
- ¼ cup cilantro, chopped
- 1 ½ cups cheddar cheese, shredded
- 1 cup pico de gallo
- 1 cup sweet corn
- 7-oz can low-sodium black beans, drained
- 3 bell peppers, cut in half & seeds removed
- ¼ tsp onion powder
- ½ tsp garlic powder
- ½ tsp chili powder
- 1 tsp adobo seasoning
- Pepper
- Salt

Directions:

Cook quinoa according to the packet instructions. Fluff quinoa with a fork and transfer to a large bowl.

Add the remaining ingredients except bell pepper into the quinoa and mix everything well.

Stuff bell peppers with quinoa mixture and place onto a baking sheet.

Bake at 360° F for 25 minutes.

Serve and enjoy.

Nutritional Data: 723 calories | 68.46g carbs | 40.52g fat | 30.22g protein | 977mg sodium

3-Grilled Chicken Caesar Salad

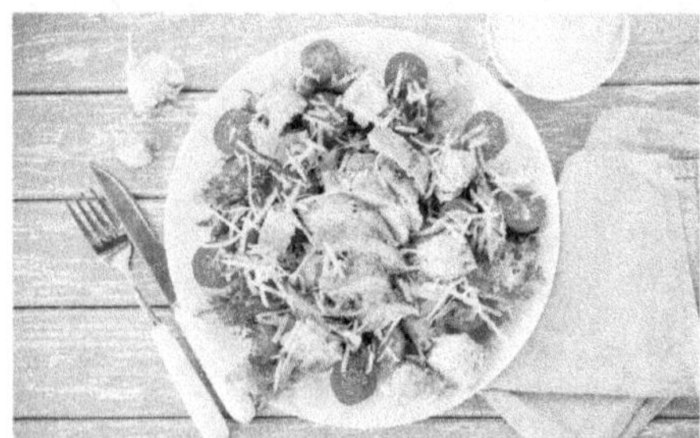

Preparation Time: 10 minutes
Cooking Time: 15 minutes
Serves: 2
Ingredients:

- 2 chicken breasts, boneless & skinless
- 2 tbsp Caesar dressing
- 1/3 cup parmesan cheese, grated
- 2 heads romaine lettuce, chopped
- 1 tbsp olive oil
- 2 sourdough bread slices, cut into pieces
- Pepper
- Salt

Directions:

Preheat broiler to high.

Arrange bread cubes on the baking sheet and broil for 3 minutes, turn the bread cubes to the other side and broil for 3 minutes more.

Preheat grill to high heat.

Brush chicken with oil and season with pepper and salt.

Arrange chicken on hot grill and cook for 4–6 minutes on each side or until internal temperature reaches 165° F.

Transfer chicken to a cutting board and cut into slices.

In a mixing bowl, add chicken, parmesan cheese, lettuce, and bread pieces.

Drizzle dressing over salad and toss well.

Serve and enjoy.

Nutritional Data: 522 calories | 29.72g carbs | 27.48g fat | 42.93g protein | 704mg sodium

4-Turkey and Avocado Wrap

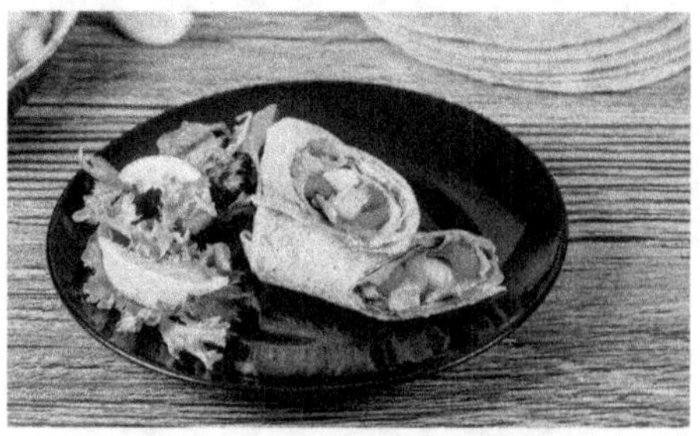

Preparation Time: 10 minutes
Cooking Time: 5 minutes
Serves: 2
Ingredients:

- 2 whole-wheat tortillas
- ½ avocado, sliced
- 1 cup green lettuce
- 1 tomato, sliced
- 1/3 lb deli turkey, sliced
- 1 tsp Cajun seasoning
- 1/8 tsp hot sauce
- ¼ cup mayonnaise

Directions:

In a small bowl, mix together mayonnaise, hot sauce, and Cajun seasoning.

Spread a tablespoon of the mayonnaise mixture on each tortilla then arrange half the turkey slices in the center of each tortilla, followed by half of the avocado, lettuce, and tomato.

Roll up the wrap tightly and secure it with a toothpick.

Serve and enjoy.

Nutritional Data: 397 calories | 31.44g carbs | 23.19g fat | 17.27g protein | 1461mg sodium

5-Vegetable Stir-Fry with Brown Rice

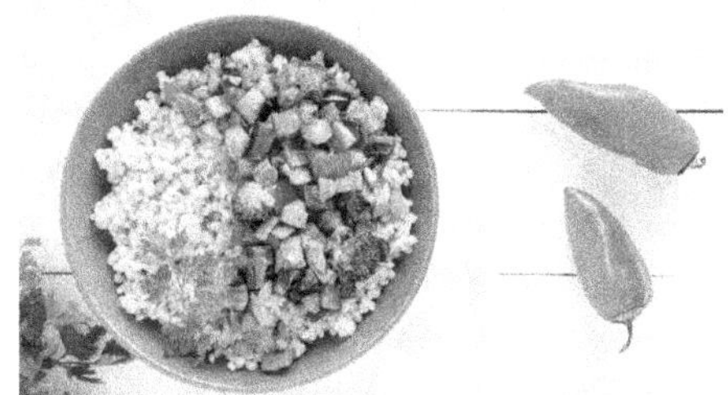

Preparation Time: 10 minutes
Cooking Time: 35 minutes
Serves: 4
Ingredients:

- ½ cup brown rice, uncooked
- 2 tbsp low-sodium soy sauce
- 1/8 tsp cayenne
- ¼ cup parsley, chopped
- 1 tbsp garlic, minced
- 2 tbsp olive oil
- ½ zucchini, chopped
- ½ bell pepper, chopped
- ½ broccoli head, chopped
- 1 cup red cabbage, chopped

Directions:

Cook rice according to the packet instructions.

Add some water in a pan and bring to a boil. Add vegetables and cook for 2 minutes over high heat. Drain vegetables and set aside.

Heat oil in the wok over medium-high heat.

Add garlic, parsley, and cayenne and cook over high heat for 1 minute.

Add rice, vegetables, and soy sauce and cook for 1–2 minutes more.

Serve and enjoy.

Nutritional Data: 194 calories | 25.54g carbs | 8.99g fat | 3.34g protein | 211mg sodium

6-Salmon and Quinoa Salad

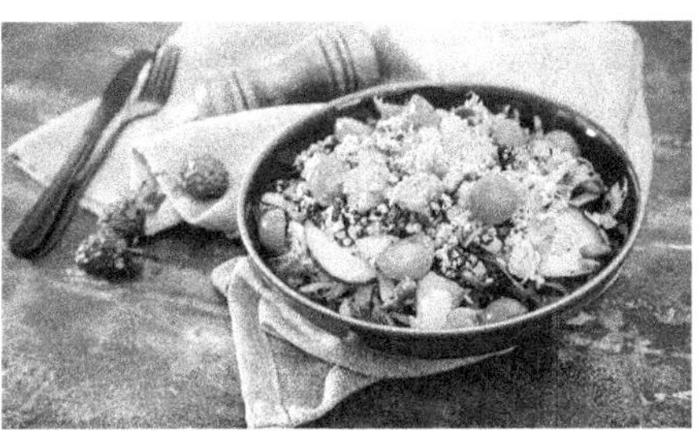

Preparation Time: 10 minutes
Cooking Time: 30 minutes
Serves: 4
Ingredients:

- 1 cup quinoa, rinsed & drained
- ¼ cup parsley, minced
- ¼ cup onion, chopped
- ½ cup cherry tomatoes, halved
- 1 lb salmon fillets
- 1 tbsp olive oil
- Pepper
- Salt
- For dressing:
- ¼ cup olive oil
- ¼ cup red wine vinegar

Directions:

Preheat the oven to 375° F.

Brush salmon with 1 tablespoon of olive oil and season with pepper and salt.

Place salmon on baking dish and bake in preheated oven for 15–20 minutes. Remove from oven and allow to cool.

Cook quinoa according to the packet instructions. Transfer cooked quinoa to a large mixing bowl. Add onion, tomatoes, and parsley, mix well, and set aside.

In a small bowl, whisk olive oil and red wine vinegar. Set aside.

Flake salmon into large chunks using a fork. Transfer salmon to quinoa mixture.

Drizzle dressing over salad and toss well to combine.

Serve and enjoy.

Nutritional Data: 491 calories | 29.45g carbs | 27.65g fat | 29.83g protein | 60mg sodium

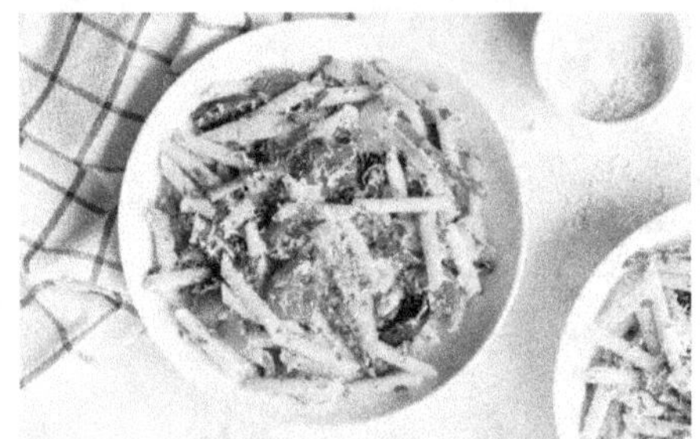

Preparation Time: 10 minutes
Cooking Time: 5 minutes
Serves: 4
Ingredients:

- 8 oz whole-wheat penne pasta
- 14-oz can tomatoes, diced
- 1/2 cup prunes
- 1/2 cup zucchini, chopped
- 1/2 cup asparagus, cut into 1-inch pieces
- 1/2 cup carrots, chopped
- 1 tbsp fresh lemon juice
- 2 tbsp fresh parsley, chopped
- 1/4 cup almonds, slivered
- 1/4 cup parmesan cheese, grated
- 1/2 cup broccoli, chopped
- 1 3/4 cups vegetable stock
- Pepper
- Salt

Directions:

Add stock, pasta, tomatoes, prunes, carrots, zucchini, asparagus, and broccoli into the instant pot and stir well.

Seal the pot with a lid and cook on high pressure for 4 minutes.

Once done, allow to release pressure manually. Remove lid.

Add remaining ingredients and stir well.

Serve and enjoy.

Nutritional Data: 226 calories | 38.85g carbs | 5.56g fat | 9.43g protein | 621mg sodium

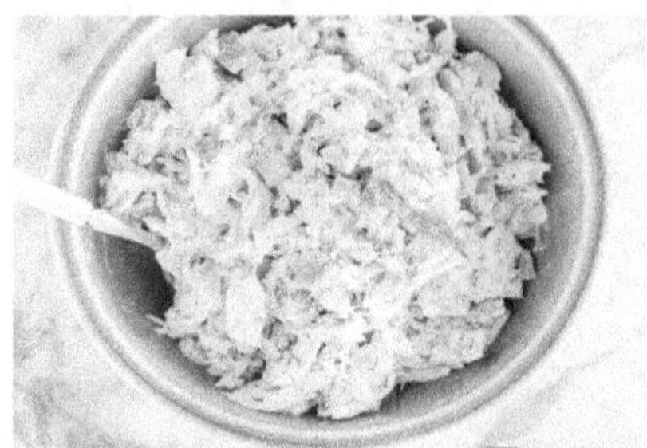

Preparation Time: 10 minutes
Cooking Time: 5 minutes
Serves: 2
Ingredients:

- 2 cups chicken, shredded
- 1 tbsp fresh parsley, chopped
- ½ tbsp Dijon mustard
- 2 tbsp almonds, chopped
- ½ cup Greek yogurt
- ¼ cup onion, chopped
- ½ cup celery, chopped
- ½ cup grapes, cut in half
- Pepper
- Salt

Directions:

Add shredded chicken and remaining ingredients to large mixing bowl and mix well.

Season salad with pepper and salt.

Serve and enjoy.

Nutritional Data: 323 calories | 12.92g carbs | 10.44g fat | 43.28g protein | 178mg sodium

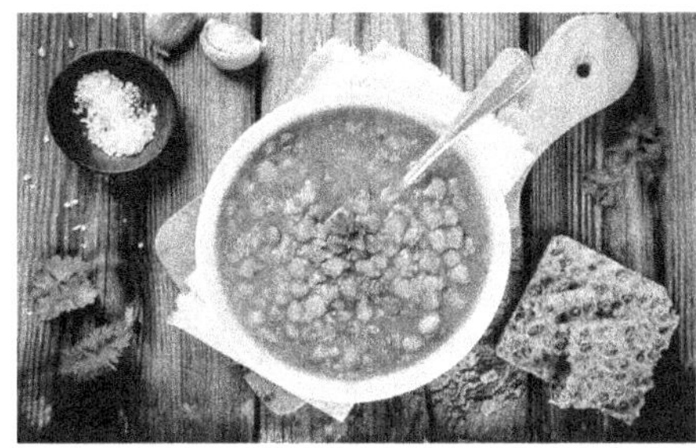

Preparation Time: 10 minutes
Cooking Time: 8 hours
Serves: 6
Ingredients:

- 2 cups dry red lentils
- 1 tbsp lemon juice
- 3 garlic cloves, minced
- 1 onion, diced
- 6 oz tomato paste
- 1/4 tsp chili powder
- 1 tsp dried thyme
- 1 tsp dried basil
- 2 tsp ground cumin
- 14-oz can tomatoes
- 3 carrots, chopped
- 6 cups vegetable stock
- Pepper
- Salt

Directions:

Add lentils and remaining ingredients into slow cooker and stir well.

Cover and cook on low for 8 hours.

Stir well and serve.

Nutritional Data: 381 calories | 69.11g carbs | 14.02g fat | 22.22g protein | 691mg sodium

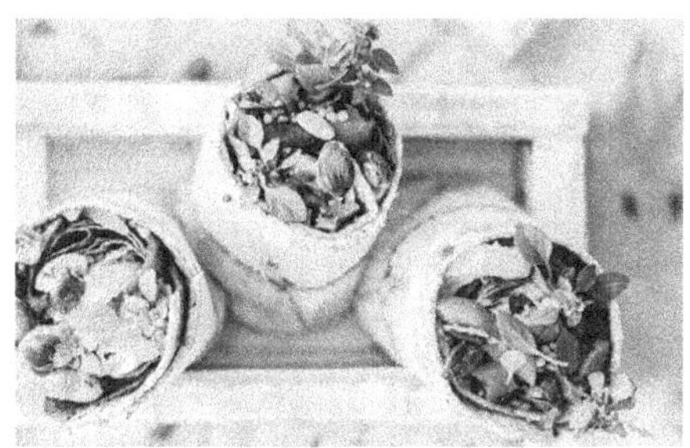

Preparation Time: 10 minutes
Cooking Time: 10 minutes
Serves: 1
Ingredients:

- 1 pita bread
- 1 1/2 cups baby greens
- 3 tablespoons hummus
- 1 teaspoon olive oil
- 2 tablespoons feta cheese, crumbled
- 6 olives, pitted & halved
- 1 medium tomato, sliced
- 1 cucumber, sliced
- Pepper
- Salt

Directions:

Spread the hummus over half of the pita bread.

Top the other half with olives, cucumber, tomatoes, onion, and baby greens.

Sprinkle with cheese and drizzle with oil. Season with pepper and salt.

Start rolling the lavash from the short end nearest the veggies until you reach the other end of the bread.

Cut the wrap in half and serve.

Nutritional Data: 552 calories | 62.13g carbs | 24.05g fat | 24.81g protein | 1690mg sodium

11-Tuna and White Bean Salad

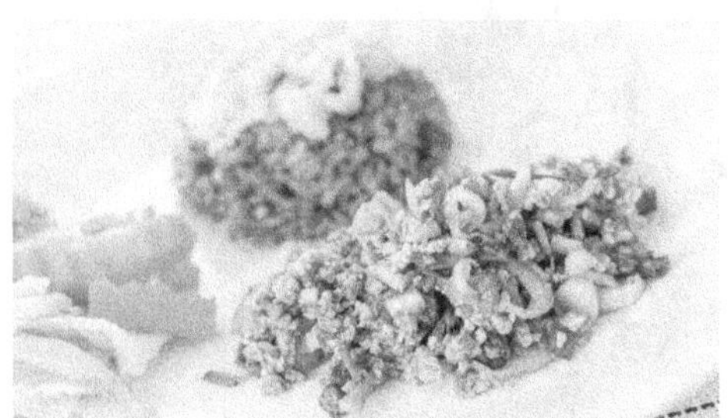

Preparation Time: 10 minutes
Cooking Time: 5 minutes
Serves: 6
Ingredients:

- 14-oz can tuna, drained
- 2 tbsp parsley, chopped
- 2 tbsp red wine vinegar
- 4 tbsp olive oil
- 1 medium onion, sliced
- 30-oz can low-sodium cannellini white beans, drained & rinsed
- Pepper
- Salt

Directions:

In a mixing bowl, mix olive oil, vinegar, pepper, and salt.

Add tuna, onion, and beans and mix well.

Garnish with parsley and serve.

Nutritional Data: 303 calories | 29.61g carbs | 10.94g fat | 22.97g protein | 504mg sodium

12-Black Bean and Corn Quesadillas

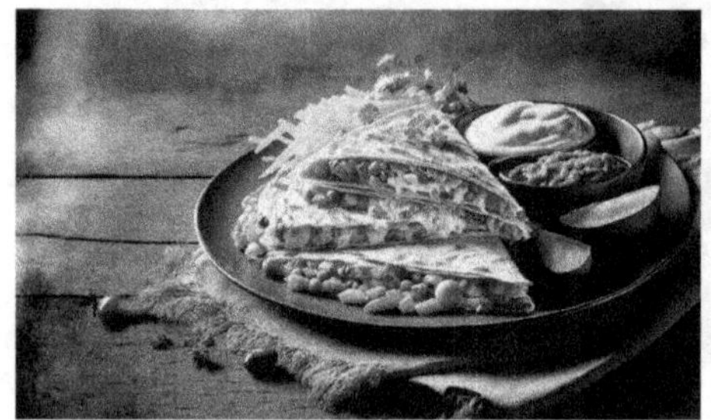

Preparation Time: 10 minutes
Cooking Time: 10 minutes
Serves: 4
Ingredients:

- 4 whole-wheat tortillas
- 15-oz can low-sodium black beans, rinsed & drained
- 1 cup sweet corn
- 2 cups Monterey jack cheese, shredded
- 2 tsp butter
- ½ tsp cumin

Directions:

In a bowl, mix black beans, cumin, and sweet corn.

Melt ½ teaspoon of butter in a pan over medium heat.

Place tortilla in the pan and add ½ cup cheese and two spoonfuls of corn-bean mixture. Fold the tortilla in half and allow to cook for 2–3 minutes on each side. Remove from the pan and repeat with the remaining tortillas.

Serve and enjoy.

Nutritional Data: 800 calories | 97.29g carbs | 27.75g fat | 44.31g protein | 794mg sodium

13-Stuffed Zucchini Boats

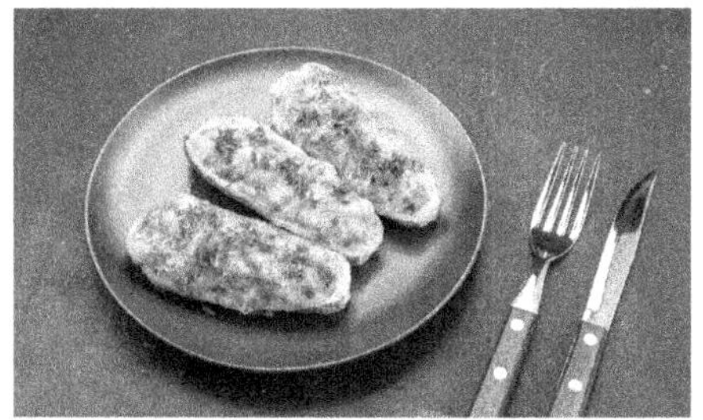

Preparation Time: 10 minutes
Cooking Time: 35 minutes
Serves: 2
Ingredients:

- 2 medium zucchinis, cut in half lengthwise & flesh scooped out using a spoon
- ½ cup mozzarella cheese, sliced
- ¼ cup parmesan cheese, grated
- ¼ tsp dried rosemary
- 1 scallion, sliced
- 2 tbsp olive oil
- ½ cup long-grain rice
- 2 tomatoes, chopped
- Pepper
- Salt

Directions:

Preheat the oven to 400° F.

Cook rice according to the packet instructions.

Heat 1 tablespoon of oil in a pan over medium-high heat.

Add zucchini flesh to the pan and cook for 5 minutes.

Add rice and scallion and mix well. Season with pepper and salt. Remove pan from heat.

Add rosemary and tomatoes and mix well.

Stuff the rice mixture into the zucchini and top with mozzarella cheese and parmesan cheese.

Bake in preheated oven for 20–25 minutes.

Serve and enjoy.

Nutritional Data: 419 calories | 46.28g carbs | 18.69g fat | 18.15g protein | 448mg sodium

14-Vegetable and Lentil Curry

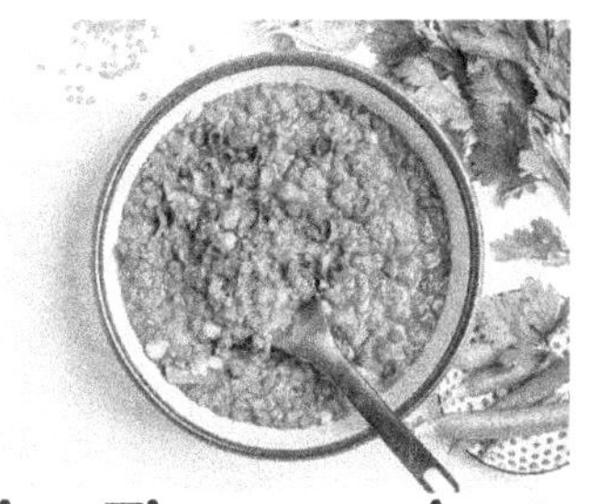

Preparation Time: 10 minutes
Cooking Time: 4 hours
Serves: 4
Ingredients:

- 1 ½ cups green lentils, rinsed
- 2 cups baby spinach
- 1/3 cup coconut milk
- 1 ½ tsp garam masala
- 1 tsp garlic, minced
- 1 tbsp ginger, minced
- 1 tbsp onion powder
- 1 tbsp olive oil
- 7 oz tomatoes, diced
- 4 cups vegetable stock
- Salt

Directions:

Add all ingredients except coconut milk and spinach into the slow cooker and mix well.

Cover and cook on high for 4 hours.

Add spinach and coconut milk and stir until spinach is wilted.

Serve and enjoy.

Nutritional Data: 215 calories | 26.16g carbs | 10.48g fat | 8.58g protein | 607mg sodium

15-Mushroom and Spinach Quesadillas

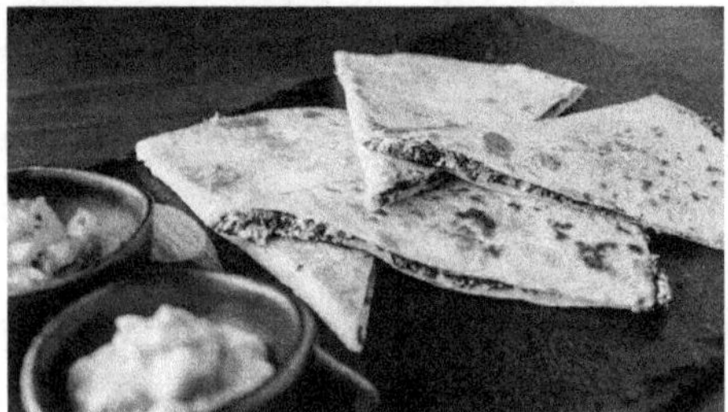

Preparation Time: 10 minutes
Cooking Time: 10 minutes
Serves: 1
Ingredients:

- 1 whole-wheat tortilla
- ¼ cup cheddar cheese, shredded
- 1 cup baby spinach
- 5 mushrooms, sliced
- 1 tbsp olive oil

Directions:

Heat oil in a pan over medium heat.

Add mushrooms and sauté until caramelized.

Add spinach and cook until wilted. Remove pan from heat.

Spray a separate pan with cooking spray and heat over medium-high heat.

Place the tortilla in the pan and layer half a side of the tortilla with the cheese and mushroom spinach mixture. Fold the tortilla in half and cook until lightly browned on both sides.

Serve and enjoy.

Nutritional Data: 185 calories | 28.38g carbs | 23.94g fat | 15.17g protein | 1007mg sodium

16-Caprese Quinoa Salad

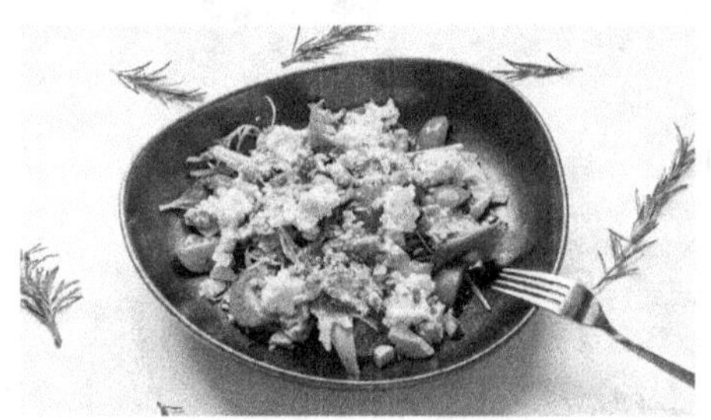

Preparation Time: 10 minutes
Cooking Time: 15 minutes
Serves: 4
Ingredients:

- 2/3 cup quinoa, rinsed
- 2 tbsp balsamic vinegar
- 2 tbsp olive oil
- ½ cup fresh basil, chopped
- 1 ½ cups cherry tomatoes, halved
- 8 oz mozzarella balls, halved
- Pepper
- Salt

Directions:

Cook quinoa according to the packet instructions. Fluff quinoa with a fork and transfer into the mixing bowl.

Add remaining ingredients into the quinoa and mix everything well.

Serve and enjoy.

Nutritional Data: 197 calories | 25.77g carbs | 8.67g fat | 4.89g protein | 60mg sodium

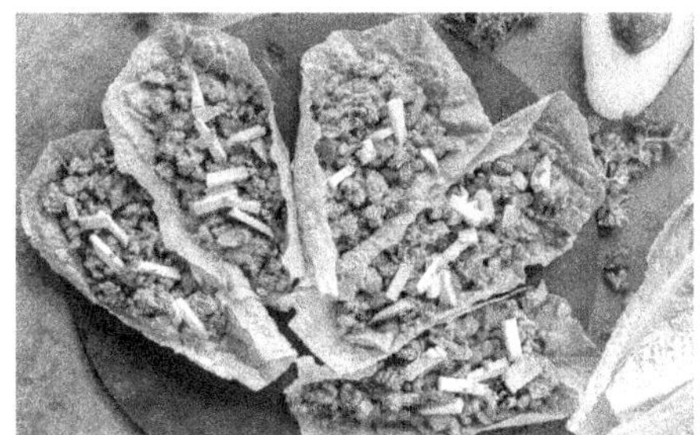

Preparation Time: 10 minutes
Cooking Time: 10 minutes
Serves: 4
Ingredients:

- 16 oz ground turkey
- ½ cup feta cheese, crumbled
- 20 cherry tomatoes, halved
- 1 large cucumber, chopped
- ½ onion, chopped
- 12 lettuce leaves
- 2 tsp garlic, minced
- 1 tbsp olive oil
- 2 tsp Greek seasoning

Directions:

Cook ground turkey in a large pan over medium heat until the meat is no longer pink.

Season with Greek seasoning and cook for 5 minutes more.

Add garlic and cook for a minute. Remove pan from heat.

Arrange lettuce leaves on a serving dish then add 2 tablespoons of the meat mixture in each of the lettuce leaves.

Top each lettuce wrap with tomatoes, cucumbers, onions, and crumbled cheese.

Serve and enjoy.

Nutritional Data: 294 calories | 11.42g carbs | 16.27g fat | 26.11g protein | 343mg sodium

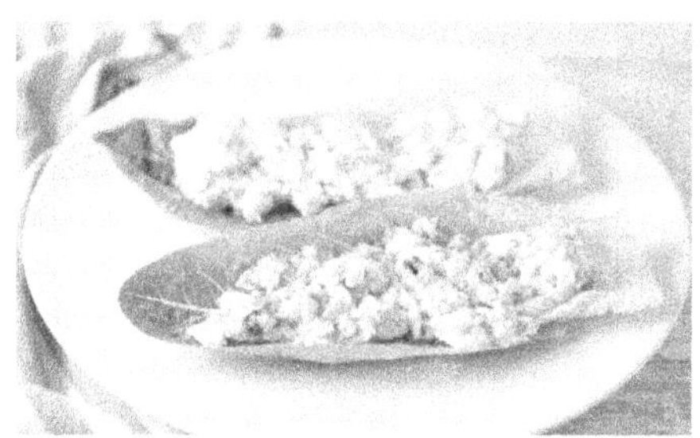

Preparation Time: 10 minutes
Cooking Time: 10 minutes
Serves: 4
Ingredients:

- 6 hard-boiled eggs, peeled & chopped
- ¼ cup mayonnaise
- 3 tbsp green onion, chopped
- 3 tbsp onion, diced
- ¼ cup celery, diced
- 1/3 cup cherry tomatoes, sliced
- Pepper
- Salt
- Lettuce leaves

Directions:

In a mixing bowl, mix chopped eggs, mayonnaise, green onion, onion, celery, and cherry tomatoes. Season with pepper and salt.

Arrange four lettuce leaves on a serving platter and add a salad on top of each leaf.

Serve and enjoy.

Nutritional Data: 175 calories | 3.62g carbs | 12.79g fat | 10.73g protein | 216mg sodium

19-Veggie and Brown Rice Sushi Rolls

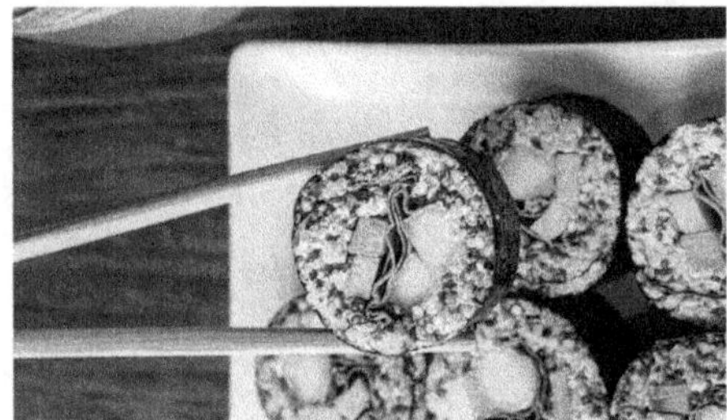

Preparation Time: 10 minutes
Cooking Time: 15 minutes
Serves: 4
Ingredients:

- 4 cups cooked sushi brown rice
- 1 cucumber, cut lengthwise
- 3 carrots, cut lengthwise
- 8 nori sheets
- ¼ cup sushi vinegar
- For sauce:
- 1 tbsp sriracha
- ¼ cup low-sodium soy sauce
- 2 tbsp sesame oil
- 3 tbsp mayonnaise

Directions:

In a small bowl, mix all sauce ingredients and set aside.

In a bowl, mix sushi rice with vinegar.

Place a nori sheet on a bamboo mat and spread 3 tablespoons of cooked sushi rice on nori.

Arrange a piece of cucumber, carrot, and 1 tablespoon of the sauce along the middle of the rice layer.

Roll the nori sheet slowly around the ingredients until you reach to other end of the roll.

Cut the roll into slices and serve.

Nutritional Data: 360 calories | 9.92g carbs | 24.37g fat | 25.81g protein | 436mg sodium

20-Sweet Potato and Black Bean Salad

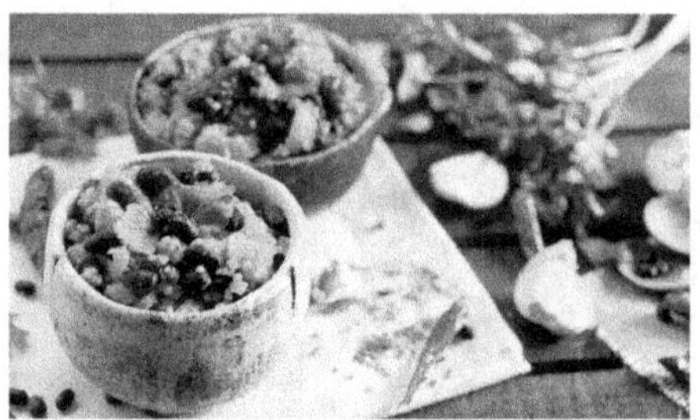

Preparation Time: 10 minutes
Cooking Time: 10 minutes
Serves: 2
Ingredients:

- 2 cups sweet potatoes, peeled & diced
- ½ cup black beans, rinsed
- 1 avocado, chopped
- 2 tbsp sunflower seeds
- 2 tbsp feta cheese, crumbled
- 1 cup cherry tomatoes, sliced
- 4 cups romaine lettuce
- 2 tbsp olive oil

Directions:

Heat olive oil in a large pan over medium heat.

Add sweet potatoes and cook for 5–8 minutes.

Divide lettuce between two serving bowls, then top it with the beans, tomatoes, sweet potatoes, avocado, sunflower seeds, and feta cheese.

Serve and enjoy.

Nutritional Data: 569 calories | 48.02g carbs | 37.09g fat | 18.51g protein | 158mg sodium

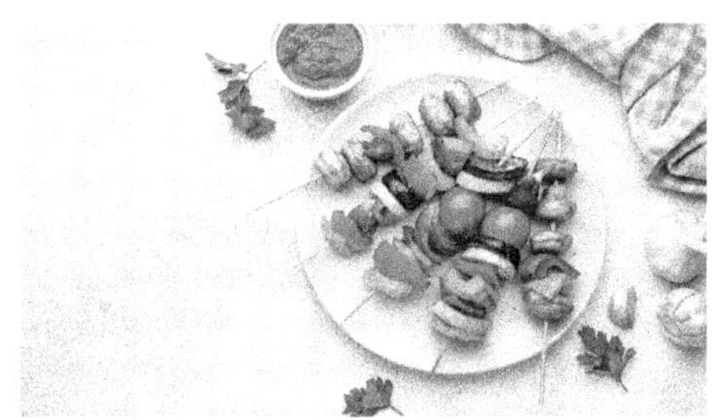

Preparation Time: 10 minutes
Cooking Time: 15 minutes
Serves: 6
Ingredients:

- 2 lbs chicken breast, cubed
- 2 cups zucchini, chopped
- 8 mushrooms, sliced
- 1/2 onion, chopped
- 6 garlic cloves, crushed
- 1/2 cup low-sodium soy sauce
- 1 bell pepper, chopped
- 4 tbsp Swerve
- 1 tsp ginger, grated

Directions:

Add chicken and remaining ingredients into a mixing bowl and mix well. Cover and place in refrigerator overnight.

Thread marinated chicken, mushrooms, zucchini, onion, and bell pepper onto the skewers.

Place chicken skewers into the air fryer basket and cook at 380° F for 15 minutes. Turn halfway through.

Serve and enjoy.

Nutritional Data: 336 calories | 8.23g carbs | 17.91g fat | 33.83g protein | 418mg sodium

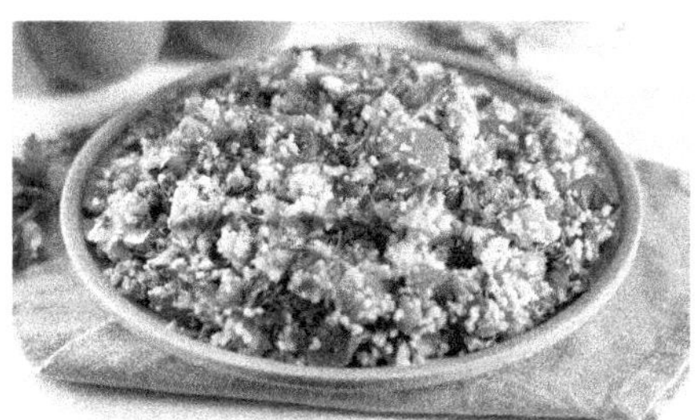

Preparation Time: 10 minutes
Cooking Time: 15 minutes
Serves: 4
Ingredients:

- 1 cup quinoa
- 2 tbsp fresh lemon juice
- 2 tbsp olive oil
- 1 tbsp parsley, chopped
- 2 tbsp olives, pitted & chopped
- ¼ cup onion, minced
- ½ cucumber, diced
- ½ cup cherry tomatoes, quartered
- 1 cup baby kale
- Pepper
- Salt

Directions:

Cook quinoa according to the packet instructions. Fluff quinoa using a fork.

Transfer cooked quinoa into large mixing bowl.

Add remaining ingredients into the quinoa and mix everything well.

Serve and enjoy.

Nutritional Data: 236 calories | 30.91g carbs | 9.91g fat | 6.73g protein | 37mg sodium

23-Black Bean and Vegetable Burrito Bowl

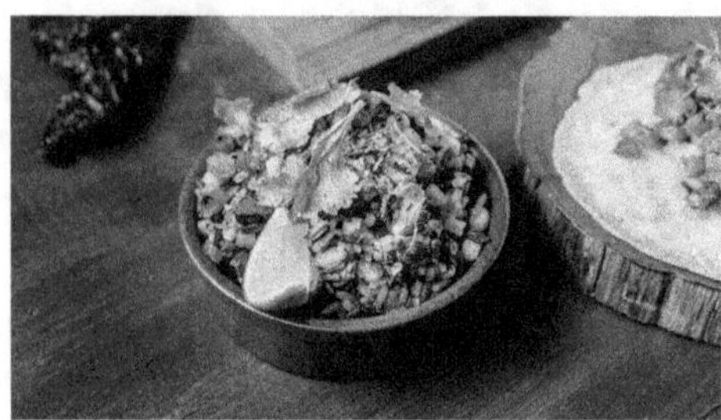

Preparation Time: 10 minutes
Cooking Time: 10 minutes
Serves: 4
Ingredients:

- For beans:
- 30-oz can low-sodium black beans, drained & rinsed
- ½ tsp cumin
- ½ tsp garlic powder
- 1 tsp oregano
- 1 tsp chili powder
- 1 tbsp lime juice
- ½ tsp salt
- For bowl:
- 3 cups cooked Mexican brown rice
- 2 cups cherry tomatoes, sliced
- 1 avocado, mashed
- 2 cups sweet corn
- 1 cup salsa
- 1 cup baby spinach

Directions:

Add black beans, cumin, garlic powder, oregano, chili powder, lime juice, and salt in a small pan and heat until the beans are warm. Remove pan from heat.

Add Mexican rice, corn, and black beans to a bowl. Top it with salsa, baby spinach, cherry tomatoes, and mashed avocado.

Serve and enjoy.

Nutritional Data: 624 calories | 84.51g carbs | 17.57g fat | 41.05g protein | 1171mg sodium

24-Mediterranean Veggie Wrap

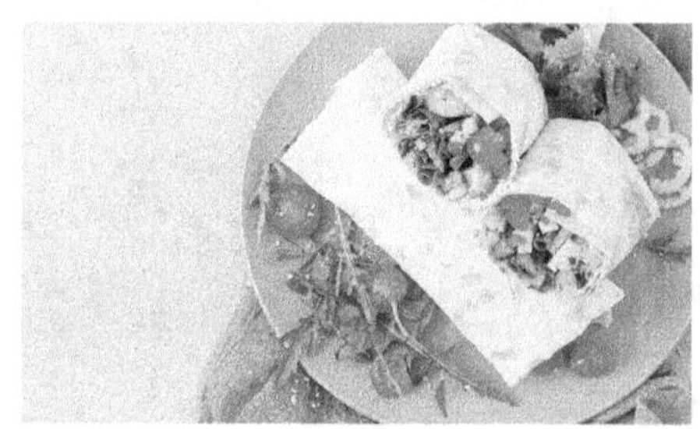

Preparation Time: 10 minutes
Cooking Time: 10 minutes
Serves: 1
Ingredients:

- 1 whole-wheat tortilla
- 6 olives, pitted & sliced
- ¼ cup cucumber, sliced
- ¼ cup roasted red peppers, sliced
- 2 lettuce leaves
- 1 tbsp feta cheese, crumbled
- 1 tbsp hummus

Directions:

Spread hummus onto the center of the tortilla then top with the feta cheese.

Add roasted peppers, cucumber, lettuce, and olives.

Roll up the wrap tightly and secure it with a toothpick.

Cut in half and serve.

Nutritional Data: 583 calories | 30.89g carbs | 39.76g fat | 26.53g protein | 1875mg sodium

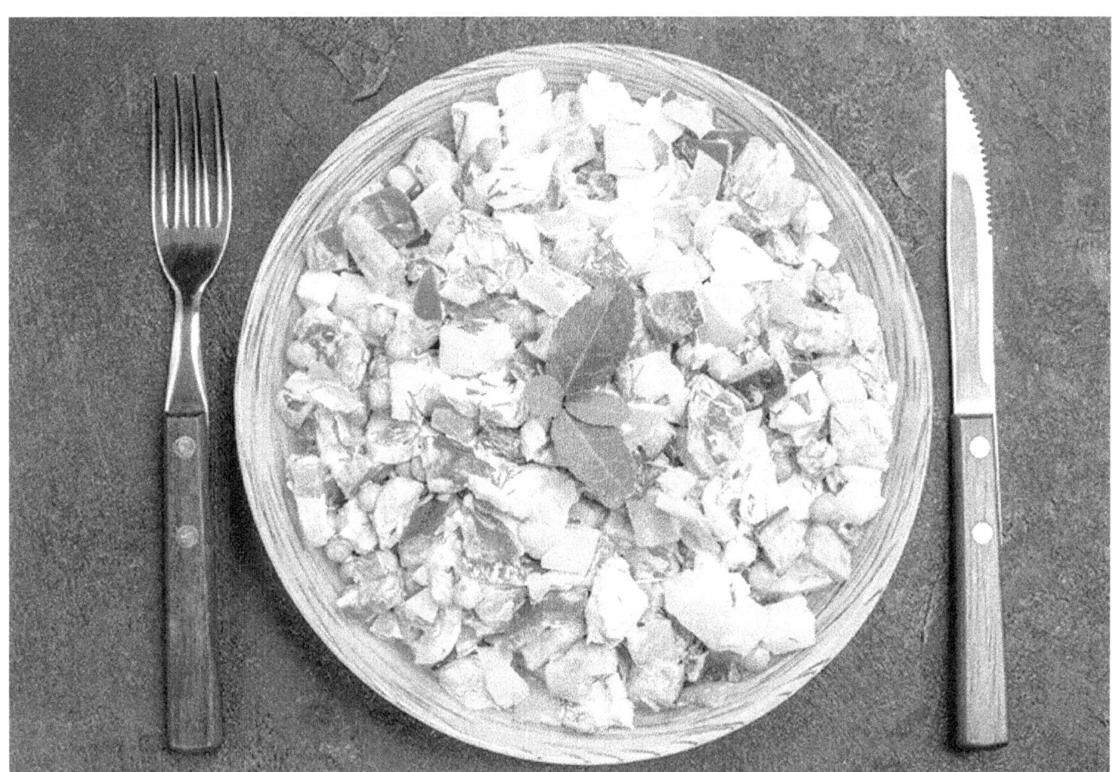

Preparation Time: 10 minutes
Cooking Time: 5 minutes
Serves: 4
Ingredients:
- 2 ½ cups sweet corn
- 1 tsp lemon juice
- 1 tbsp olive oil
- 1 avocado, cut into chunks
- 1 ½ cups cherry tomatoes, quartered
- ¼ cup parsley, chopped
- Pepper
- Salt

Directions:

In a bowl, mix sweet corn, avocado, cherry tomatoes, and parsley.

Mix together lemon juice, oil, pepper, and salt and pour over the salad.

Stir well and serve.

Nutritional Data: 234 calories | 35.18g carbs | 11.47g fat | 4.16g protein | 424mg sodium

Chapter 6 — Dinner Recipes

1-Baked Salmon with Lemon and Herbs

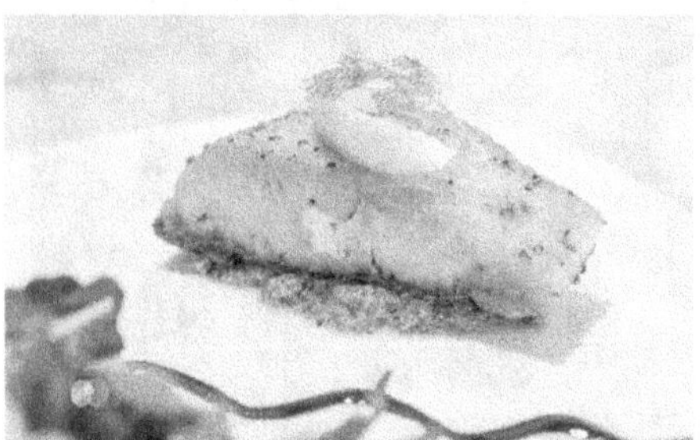

Preparation Time: 10 minutes
Cooking Time: 12 minutes
Serves: 6
Ingredients:

- 1 ½ lbs salmon fillet
- 1 tbsp lemon juice
- 1 tsp lemon zest
- 1 tsp garlic, minced
- 2 tbsp dill, chopped
- ½ tsp ground pepper
- 4 tbsp butter, melted

Directions:

Preheat the oven to 400° F.

Lightly spray a baking sheet with cooking spray and set aside.

In a small bowl, mix together butter, lemon juice, lemon zest, garlic, dill, and pepper.

Place salmon fillet skin side down onto a baking sheet. Brush salmon with butter mixture.

Bake in preheated oven for 10–12 minutes.

Serve and enjoy.

Nutritional Data: 251 calories | 1.96g carbs | 16.15g fat | 23.94g protein | 553mg sodium

2-Quinoa-Stuffed Bell Peppers

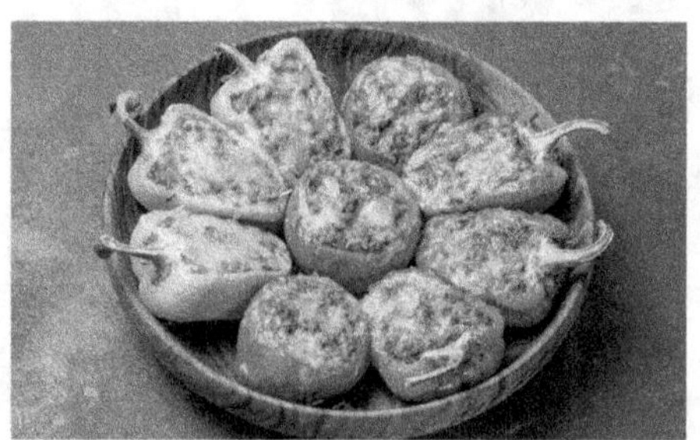

Preparation Time: 10 minutes
Cooking Time: 25 minutes
Serves: 6
Ingredients:

- 3 bell peppers, cut in half & seeds removed
- 1 tsp garlic, minced
- 1 1/2 cups cooked quinoa
- 1/3 cup chickpeas, rinsed
- 1/4 cup feta cheese, crumbled
- 1/2 cup cherry tomatoes, sliced
- 1/2 tsp oregano
- 1/2 tsp salt

Directions:

Preheat the oven to 400° F.

In a bowl, mix quinoa, oregano, garlic, tomatoes, chickpeas, and salt.

Stuff the quinoa mixture into the bell pepper halves and place onto a baking sheet.

Bake in preheated oven for 25 minutes.

Top with crumbled cheese and serve.

Nutritional Data: 181 calories | 19.29g carbs | 9g fat | 7.16g protein | 257mg sodium

3-Grilled Chicken with Roasted Vegetables

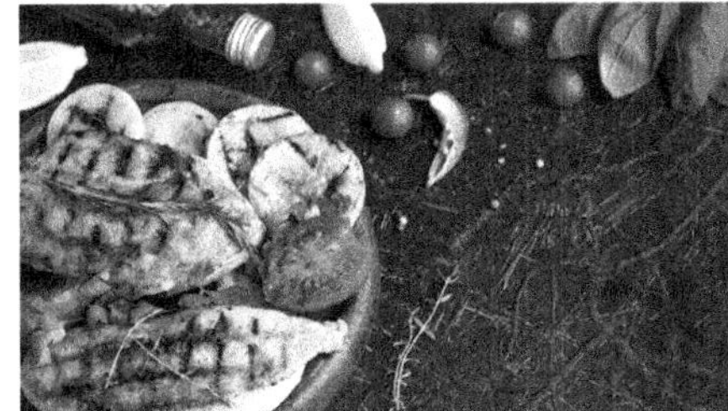

Preparation Time: 15 minutes
Cooking Time: 30 minutes
Serves: 4
Ingredients:

- 4 chicken breasts, boneless & skinless
- 2 tbsp olive oil
- Pepper
- Salt
- For Roasted vegetables:
- 1 medium onion, sliced
- 1 yellow bell pepper, cut into strips
- 1 red bell pepper, cut into strips
- 1 medium zucchini, sliced
- 1 tsp dried thyme
- 2 tbsp olive oil

Directions:

Preheat grill to medium-high heat.

Brush chicken with oil and season with pepper and salt.

Place chicken on hot grill and cook for 6–7 minutes per side or until chicken is cooked.

Preheat the oven to 425° F.

In a mixing bowl, toss onion, bell peppers, zucchini, thyme, and oil and spread over a baking sheet.

Roast vegetables in preheated oven for 20 minutes.

Slice grilled chicken and serve with roasted vegetables.

Nutritional Data: 680 calories | 7.65g carbs | 43.96g fat | 61.78g protein | 1154mg sodium

4-Turkey Chili

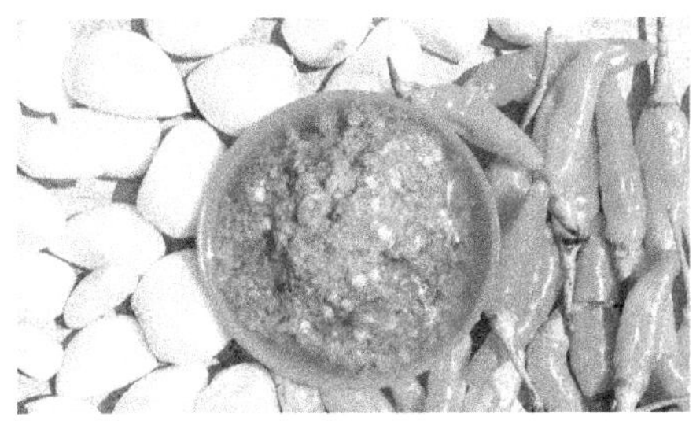

Preparation Time: 10 minutes
Cooking Time: 20 minutes
Serves: 6
Ingredients:

- 2 lbs ground turkey
- 1 sweet potato, chopped
- 3 tbsp olive oil
- 4 celery stalks, chopped
- 1 tbsp garlic, minced
- 1/2 onion, diced
- 1 tsp ginger powder
- 1 tsp cinnamon
- 1 1/3 cups pumpkin puree
- 2 cups chicken broth
- Salt

Directions:

Add oil into the instant pot and set the pot on sauté mode.

Add ground turkey and sauté until browned.

Add remaining ingredients and stir everything well.

Cover the pot with a lid and cook on high for 15 minutes.

Once done, allow to release pressure manually then open the lid carefully.

Stir well and serve.

Nutritional Data: 571 calories | 7.05g carbs | 36.77g fat | 55.26g protein | 494mg sodium

5-Lemon Garlic Shrimp with Brown Rice

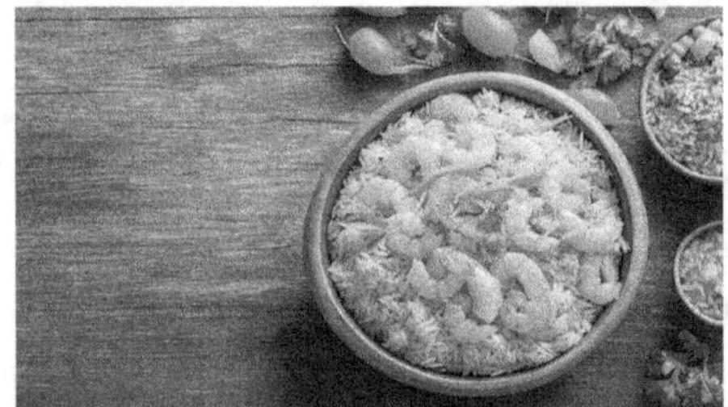

Preparation Time: 10 minutes
Cooking Time: 40 minutes
Serves: 6
Ingredients:

- 1 lb shrimp, peeled & deveined
- 2 ¼ cup vegetable stock
- 1 ½ cups brown rice
- 1 onion, chopped
- 3 tbsp parsley, chopped
- 1 tbsp garlic, minced
- 1 tsp lemon zest
- 2 tbsp lemon juice
- 3 tbsp olive oil
- Pepper
- Salt

Directions:

In a mixing bowl, mix shrimp, parsley, ½ tablespoon garlic, lemon zest, lemon juice, 2 tablespoons olive oil, pepper, and salt. Cover and let it marinate for 30 minutes.

Heat the remaining oil in a large pot over medium heat.

Add onion and garlic and sauté for 3–5 minutes.

Add brown rice and stir for a minute. Season with pepper and salt.

Add vegetable stock and bring to a boil. Turn heat to medium-low, cover and simmer for 40 minutes or until rice is tender.

Add shrimp on top of cooked rice and spread evenly. Cook shrimp for 5 minutes or until cooked.

Serve and enjoy.

Nutritional Data: 364 calories | 46.93g carbs | 9.92g fat | 21.38g protein | 1025mg sodium

6-Vegetable Stir-Fry with Tofu

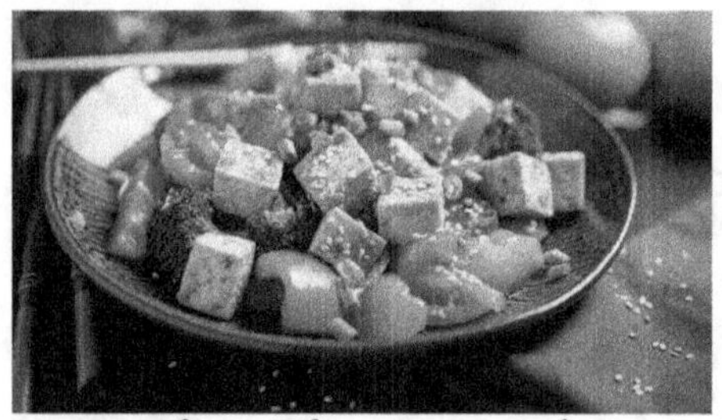

Preparation Time: 10 minutes
Cooking Time: 5 minutes
Serves: 3
Ingredients:

- 8 oz extra firm tofu, pressed and cut into cubes
- 1/4 cup onion, chopped
- 4 cherry tomatoes, chopped
- 4 cups baby spinach
- 1 tsp coconut aminos
- 3 tsp nutritional yeast
- 1/4 cup button mushrooms, chopped
- 1 tbsp olive oil

Directions:

Heat oil in a pan over medium heat.

Add onion and mushrooms and sauté until onions are softened.

Add tofu and stir for 1–2 minutes.

Add liquid aminos and nutritional yeast and stir well.

Add spinach and tomatoes and cook for 3–4 minutes.

Serve and enjoy.

Nutritional Data: 142 calories | 7.16g carbs | 9.18g fat | 10.53g protein | 218mg sodium

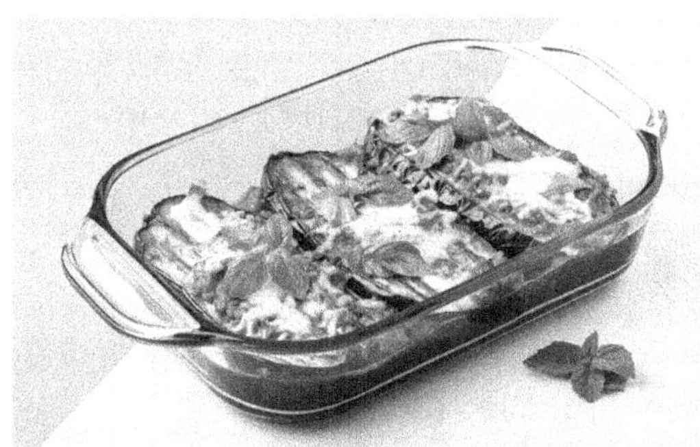

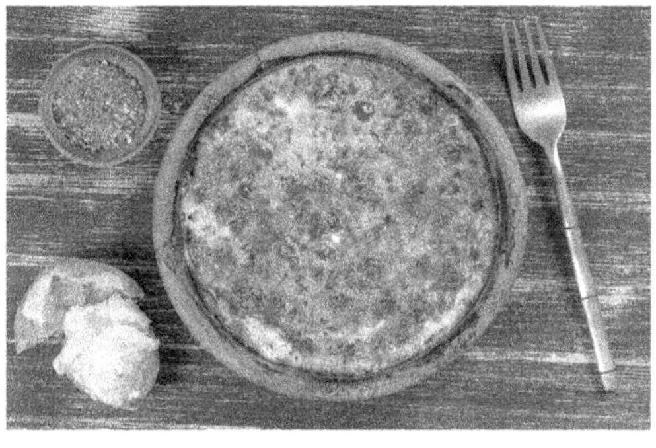

Preparation Time: 20 minutes
Cooking Time: 55 minutes
Serves: 6
Ingredients:

- 2 large eggplants, sliced
- ½ tbsp olive oil
- ¾ cup parmesan cheese, grated
- 8 oz mozzarella cheese, cut into cubes
- 1 onion, chopped
- 1 ½ lbs tomato puree
- Pepper
- Salt

Preparation Time: 15 minutes
Cooking Time: 55 minutes
Serves: 6
Ingredients:

- For pie filling:
- 14 oz cooked lentils, drained & rinsed
- ¼ cup water
- ½ tsp dried oregano
- 1 cup peas
- ¼ cup white wine
- 1 tbsp tomato puree
- 14-oz can tomatoes, chopped
- 4 oz mushrooms, chopped
- 1 carrot, chopped
- 1 bay leaf
- 1 tbsp garlic, minced
- 1 onion, chopped
- 2 tbsp olive oil
- Pepper
- Salt
- For mashed potato:
- 2 ¼ lbs potatoes, peeled & diced
- 2 tbsp butter
- 1 cup unsweetened almond milk
- Pepper
- Salt

Directions:

Add eggplant slices into colander and sprinkle with salt. Set aside for 1 hour to drain excess water.

Heat olive oil in a pan over medium heat.

Directions:

Heat olive oil in a pan over medium heat.

Add onion, garlic, and bay leaf and sauté until onion is softened.

Add mushrooms and carrots and sauté for

Add onion to the pan and sauté until softened.

Add tomato puree and stir well. Season with pepper and salt. Simmer over low heat for 10–15 minutes. Remove from heat and set aside.

Rinse the eggplant slices and pat dry with a paper towel and fry in vegetable oil for a few seconds on each side, then transfer fried eggplant slices onto the kitchen paper to remove excess oil.

Preheat oven to 350° F.

Spread a small amount of tomato sauce in a 10x8-inch baking dish. For the first layer, arrange some eggplant slices into the baking dish then top with some parmesan cheese, mozzarella cheese, and some tomato sauce. Continue the same step until the top layer is left.

For the final layer, spread the remaining tomato sauce, parmesan cheese, and mozzarella cheese.

Cover the dish with foil and bake in preheated oven for 20 minutes. Remove foil and bake for 20 minutes more.

Remove the baking dish from the oven and allow to cool for 5 minutes.

Serve and enjoy.

Nutritional Data: 215 calories | 26.41g carbs | 5.21g fat | 19.55g protein | 543mg sodium

5 minutes.

Add tomato puree, tomatoes, and white wine and cook for 5 minutes, stir constantly until the alcohol evaporates.

Add lentils, seasonings, peas, and water, and cook over low heat for 15 minutes.

For mashed potatoes: Add potatoes into a pot, cover with water, and cook until potatoes are tender.

Once potatoes are cooked, drain the water. Add butter and milk to the potatoes and mash until smooth and creamy. Season with pepper and salt.

•Preheat the oven to 390° F.

•Add lentil mixture into a baking dish then spread mashed potatoes on top of the lentil mixture evenly.

•Bake in preheated oven for 20 minutes.

•Serve and enjoy.

Nutritional Data: 437 calories | 79.21g carbs | 9.76g fat | 14.08g protein |163mg sodium

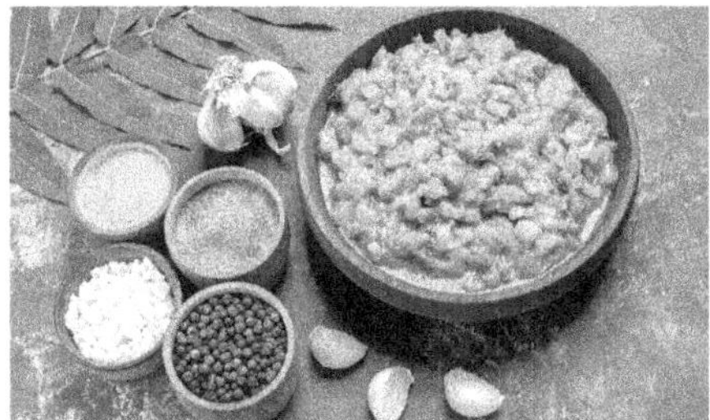

Preparation Time: 10 minutes
Cooking Time: 8 hours
Serves: 6
Ingredients:

- 2 cups dried brown lentils
- 14 oz coconut milk
- 3 cups vegetable broth
- 14 oz potatoes, diced
- 3 tbsp curry powder
- 14 oz tomatoes, diced
- 1 medium sweet potato, peeled & diced
- 2 large carrots, peeled & sliced
- 1 tbsp garlic, minced
- 1 onion, diced
- Pepper
- Salt

Directions:

Add lentils, broth, potatoes, curry powder, tomatoes, sweet potato, carrots, garlic, onion, pepper, and salt into slow cooker and stir well.

Cover and cook on low for 8 hours.

Add coconut milk and stir everything well.

Serve with rice and enjoy.

Nutritional Data: 289 calories | 33.72g carbs | 16.62g fat | 7.16g protein | 330mg sodium

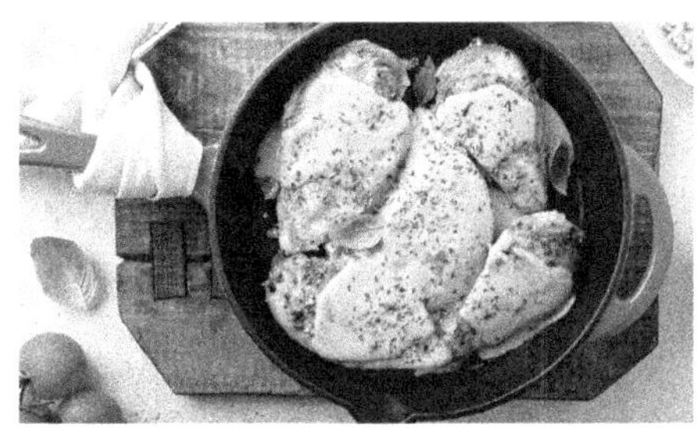

Preparation Time: 10 minutes
Cooking Time: 40 minutes
Serves: 6
Ingredients:

- 1 egg
- 2 1/2 lbs chicken breast
- 1/2 tbsp dried oregano
- 1/2 tbsp dried onion, minced
- 1/2 tbsp dried garlic, minced
- 6 oz mozzarella cheese, shredded
- 3/4 cup marinara sauce
- 1/2 tbsp dried parsley
- 1/2 tbsp dried basil
- 1 cup parmesan cheese, grated
- Salt

Directions:

Preheat the oven to 400° F.

Line baking sheet with parchment paper and set aside.

•n a small bowl, whisk the egg.

In a separate bowl, mix parmesan cheese and spices.

Dip each chicken breast in the egg then coat with cheese mixture and place onto a baking sheet.

Bake in preheated oven for 30 minutes.

Top with marinara sauce and mozzarella cheese and bake for 10 minutes more.

Serve and enjoy.

Nutritional Data: 475 calories | 6.41g carbs | 24.21g fat | 55.15g protein | 657mg sodium

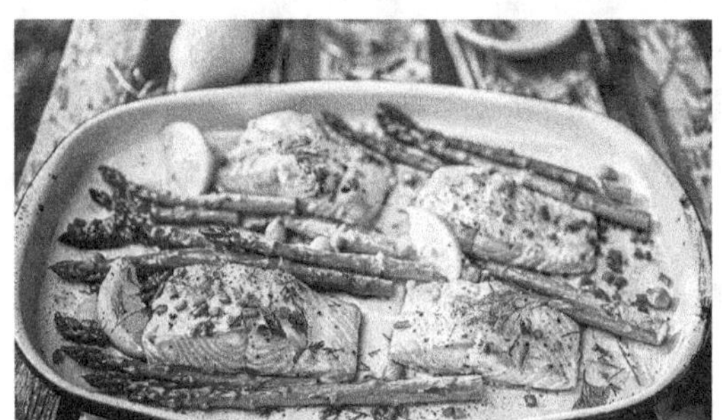

Preparation Time: 10 minutes
Cooking Time: 10 minutes
Serves: 4
Ingredients:

- 4 salmon fillets
- 1 lemon, sliced
- ½ lemon, juiced
- 3 tbsp olive oil
- 1 tbsp garlic, minced
- 1 ½ tbsp dill, chopped
- 1 ½ lb asparagus, trimmed
- Pepper
- Salt

Directions:

Preheat the oven broiler to high heat.

Arrange salmon fillets and asparagus on a baking sheet. Season with pepper and salt.

Sprinkle dill over salmon.

In a small bowl, mix oil, lemon juice, and garlic and pour over salmon and asparagus.

Arrange the lemon slices over the salmon and asparagus.

Broil in preheated oven broiler for 10 minutes.

Serve and enjoy.

Nutritional Data: 303 calories | 10.97g carbs | 18.29g fat | 26.22g protein | 460mg sodium

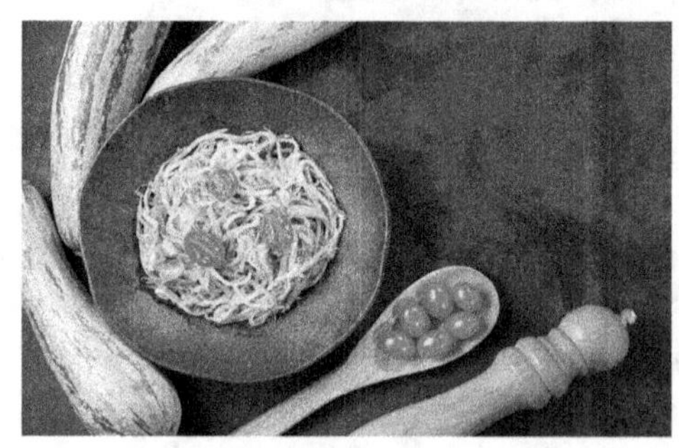

Preparation Time: 10 minutes
Cooking Time: 10 minutes
Serves: 2
Ingredients:

- 1 zucchini, spiralized
- 2 tbsp fresh lemon juice
- 1/4 cup pine nuts
- 1/3 cup water
- 3/4 cup cherry tomatoes, halved
- 1 avocado, chopped
- 1 1/4 cup fresh basil
- Pepper
- Salt

Directions:

Add zucchini noodles and cherry tomatoes into mixing bowl.

Add the remaining ingredients into blender and blend until smooth.

Pour the blended mixture over zucchini noodles.

Toss well and serve.

Nutritional Data: 293 calories | 15.03g carbs | 26.49g fat | 5.48g protein | 11mg sodium

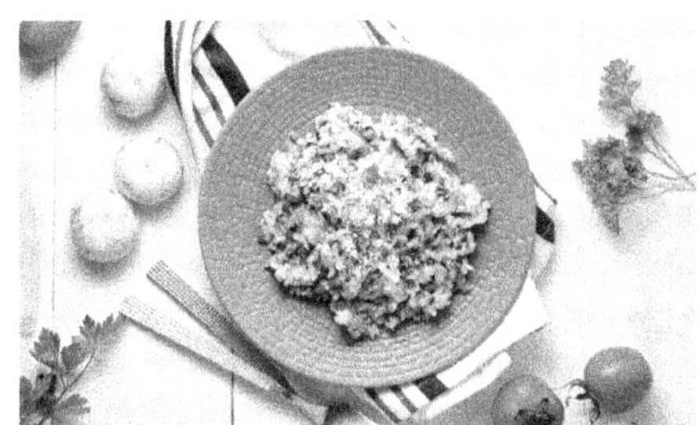

Preparation Time: 10 minutes
Cooking Time: 30 minutes
Serves: 4
Ingredients:

- 1 cup Arborio rice
- 1/3 cup spinach, chopped
- ½ cup mushrooms, sliced
- ½ cup white wine
- ¼ cup parmesan cheese, grated
- 6 cups chicken stock
- ½ cup onion, diced
- 1 tbsp olive oil
- 2 tbsp butter
- Pepper
- Salt

Directions:

Add butter and oil in a saucepan and heat over medium heat.

Add onion and mushrooms and cook until onions are translucent.

Add Arborio rice and stir for a minute.

Add white wine and cook until the wine evaporates.

Add stock, turn heat to medium-low, and cook for 20–25 minutes or until rice is al dente.

Add spinach and stir until wilted.

Remove risotto from heat. Add parmesan cheese and stir well.

Serve and enjoy.

Nutritional Data: 343 calories | 31.08g carbs | 21.39g fat | 15.47g protein | 680mg sodium

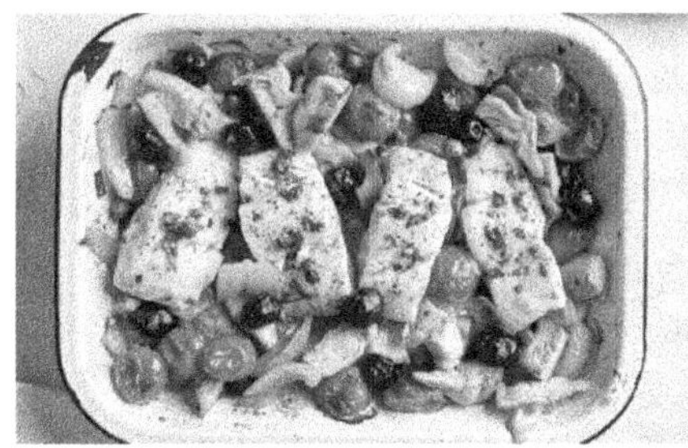

Preparation Time: 10 minutes
Cooking Time: 10 minutes
Serves: 6
Ingredients:

- 24 oz cod fillet, cut into 6 pieces
- 1 tsp dried oregano
- 1 lemon juice
- 2 tbsp onion, minced
- ¼ cup olive oil
- ¼ cup olives, chopped
- ¼ cup yellow bell pepper, diced
- 1/3 cup cucumber, diced
- 1/3 cup tomatoes, diced
- Pepper
- Salt

Directions:

Preheat the oven to 400° F.

Arrange cod pieces onto a baking sheet. Brush with 1 tablespoon of oil and season with oregano, pepper, and salt.

Bake in preheated oven for 10–12 minutes or until internal temperature reaches 145° F.

Meanwhile for salsa, in a mixing bowl, mix tomatoes, olives, onion, cucumber, and yellow pepper. Mix together remaining oil, lemon juice, pepper, and salt and pour over the salsa. Mix well.

Add salsa on top of each cooked cod piece and serve.

Nutritional Data: 174 calories | 2.68g carbs | 10.14g fat | 17.74g protein | 386mg sodium

15-Stuffed Acorn Squash

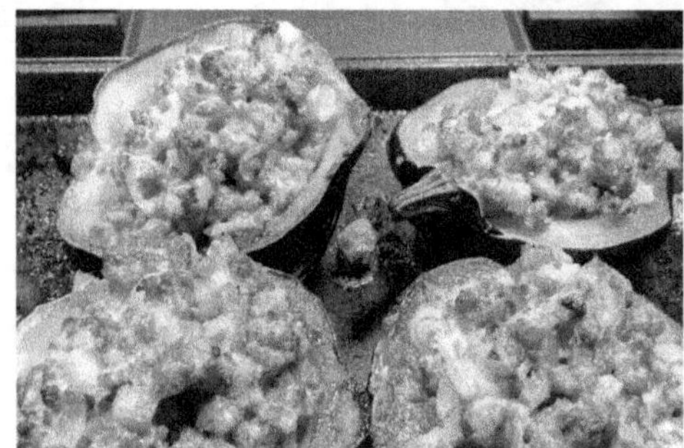

Preparation Time: 10 minutes
Cooking Time: 30 minutes
Serves: 4
Ingredients:

- 2 small acorn squash, cut in half & seeds removed
- 1/3 cup roasted pistachios, chopped
- 1/3 cup feta cheese, crumbled
- 2 tbsp chives, chopped
- ½ cup quinoa, rinsed & drained
- 1 lemon, juiced
- 2 garlic cloves, minced
- 1 ½ cups water
- 2 tbsp olive oil
- Pepper
- Salt

Directions:

Preheat the oven to 400° F.

Line baking sheet with parchment paper and set aside.

Brush the cut side of the squash with oil and season with pepper and salt.

Place squash cut side down on the baking sheet and bake in preheated oven for 25–30 minutes.

16-Turkey Meatballs with Marinara Sauce

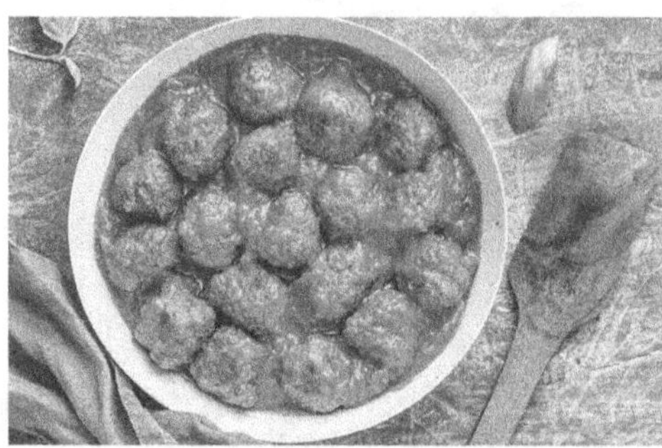

Preparation Time: 10 minutes
Cooking Time: 45 minutes
Serves: 18
Ingredients:

- 1 egg
- 1 lb ground turkey
- 1/8 tsp red pepper flakes, crushed
- 2 garlic cloves, minced
- 1 tbsp Italian seasoning
- ½ cup parmesan cheese, grated
- ½ onion, diced
- ¼ cup almond flour
- Pepper
- Salt
- For marinara sauce:
- 28 oz crushed tomatoes
- ½ tsp dried oregano
- 1 tsp dried basil
- 1 tbsp garlic, minced
- ½ cup onion, diced
- Pepper
- Salt

Directions:

Spray a small saucepan with cooking spray and heat over medium heat.

Add onion and garlic and sauté for 1–2 minutes.

Add tomatoes, basil, oregano, pepper, and salt and stir well. Cook over low heat for 10–15 minutes. Remove from heat and set aside.

For meatballs: Preheat the oven to 350°

Add water, lemon juice, and garlic in a saucepan and bring to a boil.

Add quinoa, turn the heat to medium-low, and cook for 15 minutes or until all liquid is absorbed. Remove from heat and allow to cool for 15 minutes.

Fluff quinoa with a fork and transfer to a mixing bowl. Add parsley, pistachios, feta cheese, chives, pepper, and salt, and stir well to combine.

Stuff filling into the baked squash and serve immediately.

Nutritional Data: 324 calories | 41.84g carbs | 15.57g fat | 8.95g protein | 124mg sodium

F.

Lightly grease the baking sheet with cooking spray and set aside.

In a mixing bowl, add all meatball ingredients and mix until well combined.

Make equal shapes of balls from the meat mixture and place onto a baking sheet and bake in preheated oven for 25–30 minutes.

Toss meatballs in marinara sauce and serve.

Nutritional Data: 74 calories | 3.94g carbs | 3.44g fat | 7.09g protein | 147mg sodium

17-Eggplant and Zucchini Lasagna

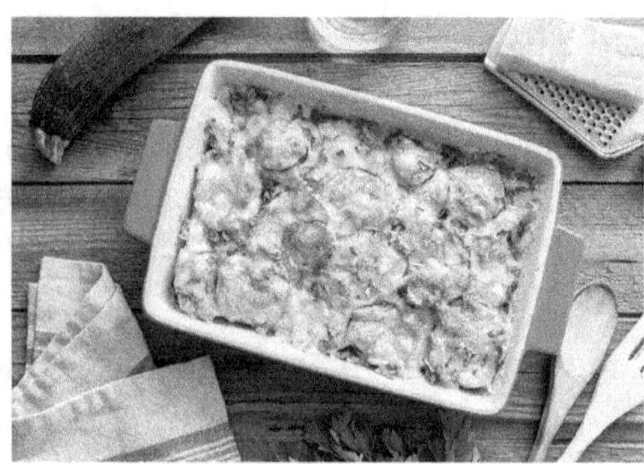

Preparation Time: 10 minutes
Cooking Time: 55 minutes
Serves: 6
Ingredients:

- 1 egg
- 2 cups mozzarella cheese, shredded
- 24 oz marinara sauce
- ¼ cup parmesan cheese, grated
- 15 oz ricotta cheese
- 2 tbsp olive oil
- 1 medium eggplant, cut into ¼-inch thick slices

2 large zucchinis, cut into ¼-inch thick slices

Directions:

Preheat the oven to 400° F.

Lightly grease two baking sheets with cooking spray.

Arrange eggplant and zucchini slices onto a baking sheet and drizzle with oil.

Bake in preheated oven for 12 minutes.

In a mixing bowl, mix ricotta cheese, 2 tablespoons of parmesan cheese, and egg until well combined. Set aside.

18-Black Bean and Sweet Potato Tacos

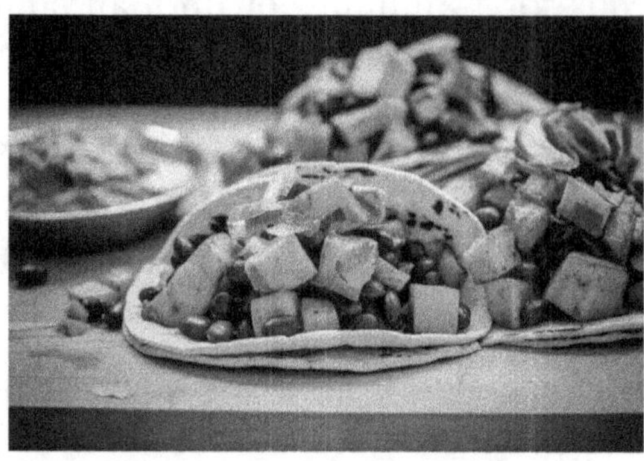

Preparation Time: 10 minutes
Cooking Time: 28 minutes
Serves: 5
Ingredients:

- 1 ½ lbs sweet potatoes, peeled & diced into ½-inch cubes
- 2 tbsp fresh cilantro, chopped
- 3 tbsp lime juice
- 3 tbsp honey
- 1 cup corn
- 14-oz can black beans, drained & rinsed
- 1 ½ tsp garlic, minced
- 1 cup onion, diced
- ½ tsp ground coriander
- 1 tsp paprika
- 1 tsp cumin
- 4 tbsp olive oil
- Pepper
- Salt

Directions:

Preheat the oven to 425° F.

Line baking sheet with parchment paper.

Arrange sweet potatoes onto a baking sheet and drizzle with 3 tablespoons of olive oil. Toss well to coat.

Season with cumin, coriander, paprika, pepper, and salt, and toss to coat evenly. Bake in preheated oven for 20 minutes or until tender. Remove from oven.

Spread ½ cup marinara sauce in the bottom of 8x8-inch baking dish. Layer 1/3 of the zucchini slices, 1/3 of the eggplant slices, then ½ cup marinara sauce, and ½ of the ricotta mixture. Top with 2/3 cup mozzarella cheese. Repeat.

Cover the baking dish with foil and bake in preheated oven for 30 minutes. Remove foil and bake for 10 minutes more. Remove from oven and allow to cool for 10 minutes.

Serve and enjoy.

Nutritional Data: 352 calories | 21.48g carbs | 18.65g fat | 26.4g protein | 917mg sodium

Heat the remaining olive oil in a pan over medium-high heat.

Add onion and sauté for 5 minutes. Add garlic and sauté for 30 seconds.

Add black beans, lime juice, honey, and corn, and cook over medium-low heat until just warm.

Toss in sweet potatoes and serve over tortillas.

Nutritional Data: 436 calories | 70.35g carbs | 13.7g fat | 14.26g protein | 24mg sodium

19-Spinach and Mushroom-Stuffed Chicken Breast

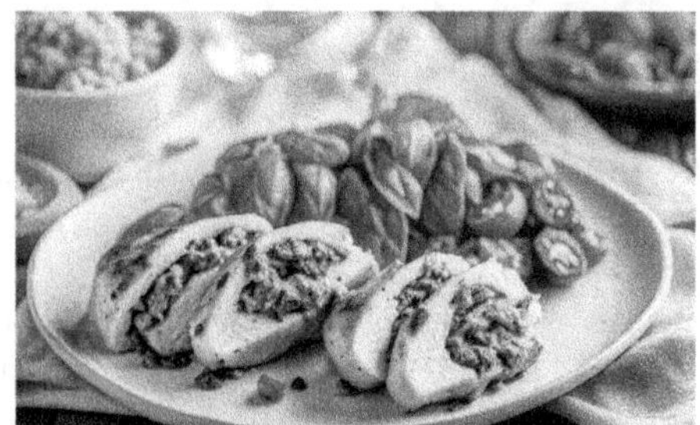

Preparation Time: 10 minutes
Cooking Time: 15 minutes
Serves: 3
Ingredients:

- 3 chicken breasts, skinless & boneless, sliced in half without slicing them all the way through
- ¾ cup mozzarella cheese, grated
- 2 cups spinach, chopped
- ½ tsp Italian seasoning
- 10 mushrooms, sliced
- 2 garlic cloves, minced
- 1 tsp butter
- 2 tbsp olive oil
- Pepper
- Salt

Directions:

Heat a tablespoon of olive oil in a pan over medium heat.

Add garlic, mushrooms, Italian seasoning, and salt, and cook over high heat for 2–3 minutes. Transfer mushrooms to a bowl and set aside.

Season chicken with pepper and salt. Stuff each chicken breast with mushrooms, spinach, and cheese and secure with a toothpick.

Heat butter and remaining oil in a pan over medium heat. Place stuffed chicken breasts into the pan and cook for 6–7 minutes on each side.

Serve and enjoy.

Nutritional Data: 649 calories | 4.72g carbs | 37.28g fat | 71.08g protein | 455mg sodium

20-Lemon Herb Chicken Skewers

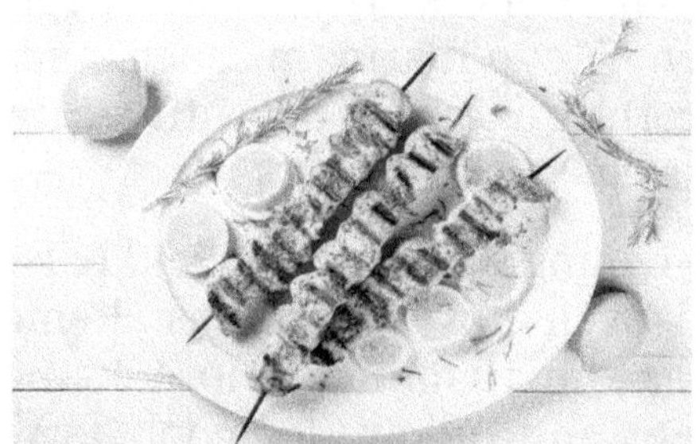

Preparation Time: 10 minutes
Cooking Time: 10 minutes
Serves: 4
Ingredients:

- 1 1/2 lbs chicken breast, cut into 1-inch cubes
- For marinade:
- 1/2 cup lemon juice
- 1/4 tsp cayenne
- 2 tbsp fresh rosemary, chopped
- 2 tbsp dried oregano
- 1/2 cup yogurt
- 1 tbsp red wine vinegar
- 4 garlic cloves
- 1/4 cup fresh mint leaves
- 1 cup olive oil
- Pepper
- Salt

Directions:

Add all marinade ingredients into the blender and blend until smooth.

Pour the blended mixture into a bowl.

Add chicken to the bowl and coat well.

Cover and place in refrigerator for 1 hour.

Preheat the grill over medium-high heat.

Remove the marinated chicken from the refrigerator and thread onto the skewers.

Place skewers on the hot grill and cook for 5–7 minutes on each side or until the chicken is cooked.

Serve and enjoy.

Nutritional Data: 809 calories | 6.3g carbs | 70.95g fat | 37.27g protein | 125mg sodium

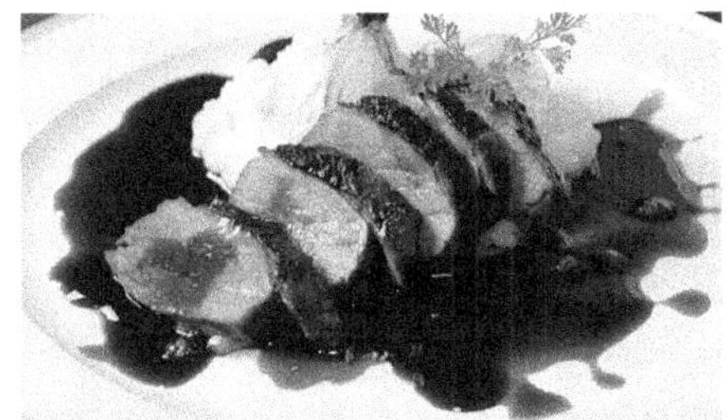

Preparation Time: 10 minutes
Cooking Time: 30 minutes
Serves: 4
Ingredients:

- 2 ½ lbs pork tenderloin
- 2 tbsp canola oil
- For glaze:
- 2 tsp balsamic vinegar
- 1 tbsp olive oil
- 3 tbsp Dijon mustard
- ½ cup apple cider vinegar glaze
- Pepper
- Salt

Directions:

Preheat the oven to 350° F.

Line baking sheet with parchment paper and set aside.

In a small bowl, mix together all glaze ingredients and set aside.

Season pork tenderloin with pepper and salt.

Heat canola oil in a large pan over medium-high heat. Place pork in a pan and sear for 2–3 minutes on each side.

Brush pork with half the glaze and cook in preheated oven for 30 minutes. Brush pork with remaining glaze and cook for 20 minutes more or until internal temperature reaches 150° F. Remove from oven and let it cool for 10 minutes before serving.

Slice and serve.

Nutritional Data: 525 calories | 5.7g carbs | 20.78g fat | 74.9g protein | 293mg sodium

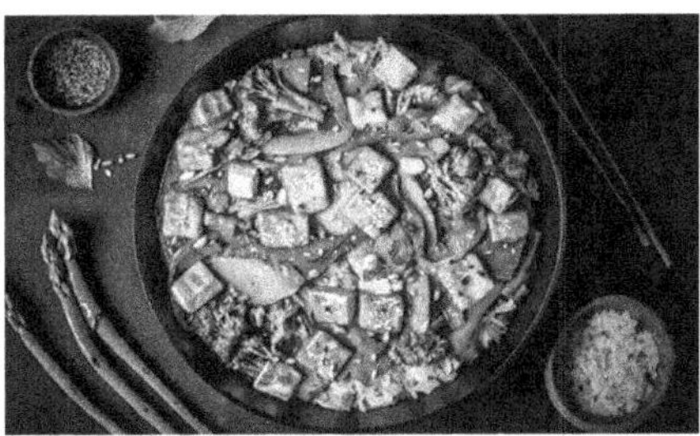

Preparation Time: 10 minutes
Cooking Time: 10 minutes
Serves: 4
Ingredients:

- 8 oz extra-firm tofu, cut into 1-inch pieces
- 2 tbsp olive oil
- 6 oz mushrooms, sliced
- 1/2 tbsp rice vinegar
- 1 tbsp low-sodium soy sauce
- 3 baby bok choy, sliced
- 3 garlic cloves, minced
- Pepper
- Salt

Directions:

Heat olive oil in a pan over medium heat.

Add garlic and sauté for a minute.

Add tofu and mushrooms and stir fry for 3–5 minutes.

Add bok choy and stir fry for 2 minutes.

Add soy sauce, vinegar, pepper, and salt, and stir everything well.

Serve and
enjoy.

Nutritional Data: 317 calories | 48.01g carbs | 12.16g fat | 11.28g protein | 99mg sodium

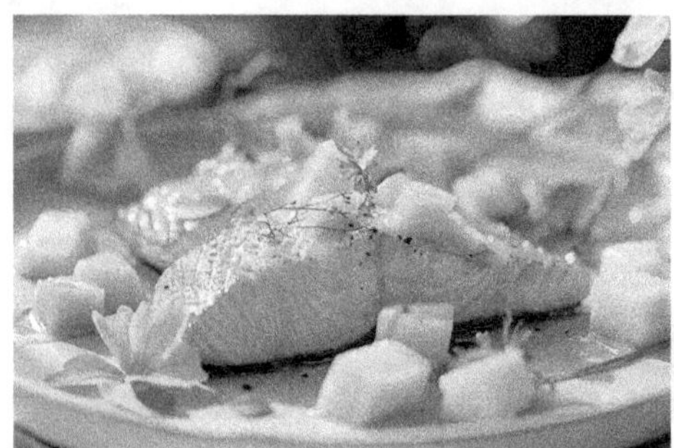

Preparation Time: 10 minutes
Cooking Time: 15 minutes
Serves: 4
Ingredients:

- 4 salmon fillets
- 2 tbsp honey
- 2 tbsp butter
- 2 tsp olive oil
- Pepper
- Salt
- For salsa:
- 2 mangoes, peeled & diced
- 1 lime, juiced
- ¼ cup fresh cilantro, chopped
- ½ onion, diced
- 1 red bell pepper, diced
- Pinch of salt

Directions:

In a medium bowl, add all salsa ingredients and mix well. Set aside.

Brush salmon with oil and season with pepper and salt.

Melt butter in a pan over medium heat. Once butter is melted, add honey and stir well.

Arrange salmon fillets in a pan and cook for 4–5 minutes. Flip salmon fillets and cook for 5–8 minutes.

Top salmon with salsa and serve.

Nutritional Data: 303 calories | 20.52g carbs | 15.44g fat | 21.8g protein | 482mg sodium

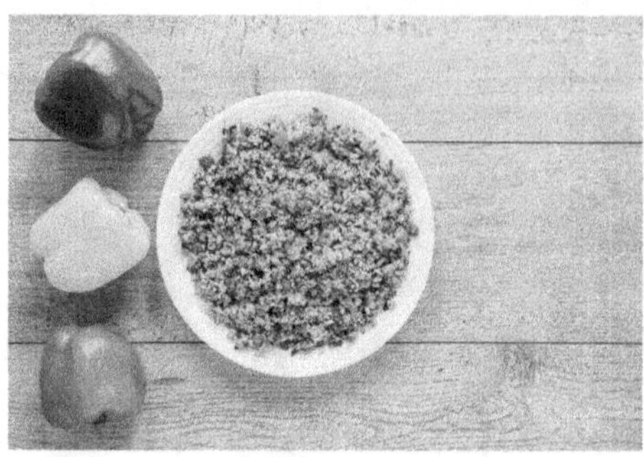

Preparation Time: 10 minutes
Cooking Time: 20 minutes
Serves: 6
Ingredients:

- 1 ½ cups quinoa, rinsed & drained
- 1/8 tsp garlic powder
- 2 tbsp low-sodium soy sauce
- 2 cups spinach
- 8 oz mushrooms, sliced
- 3 garlic cloves, minced
- 1 tbsp olive oil
- 2 cups water
- Pepper
- Salt

Directions:

Add quinoa and water in a saucepan and cook over medium heat until all liquid evaporates, about 15 minutes.

Heat oil in a large pan over medium heat.

Add mushrooms, garlic, spinach, garlic powder, and soy sauce and cook for 3–4 minutes.

Add quinoa, stir everything well, and cook for 1 minute.

Serve and enjoy.

Nutritional Data: 641 calories | 84.13g carbs | 25.74g fat | 24.74g protein | 575mg sodium

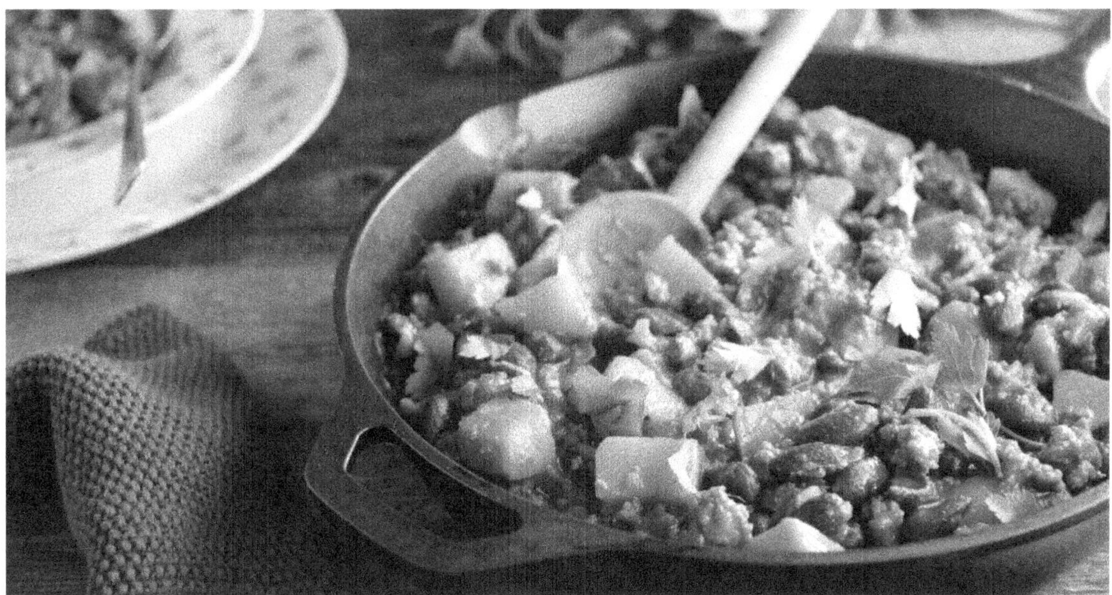

Preparation Time: 10 minutes
Cooking Time: 25 minutes
Serves: 4
Ingredients:
- 1 lb ground turkey
- ¼ cup fresh parsley, chopped
- 1 avocado, chopped
- 1 tomato, chopped
- 1 tbsp onion powder
- 1 tbsp garlic powder
- 4 oz mushrooms, sliced
- 1 bell pepper, chopped
- ½ onion, chopped
- 2 tbsp olive oil
- Pepper
- Salt

Directions:

Heat oil in a large pan over medium heat.

Add onion, mushrooms, and bell pepper and sauté until vegetables are softened.

Add ground turkey and spices and cook until meat is completely cooked through.

Top with avocado, tomatoes, and parsley. Season with pepper and salt.

Serve and enjoy.

Nutritional Data: 427 calories | 33.63g carbs | 23.27g fat | 27.58g protein | 82mg sodium

Chapter 7 — Dessert Recipes

1-Frozen Yogurt Bark

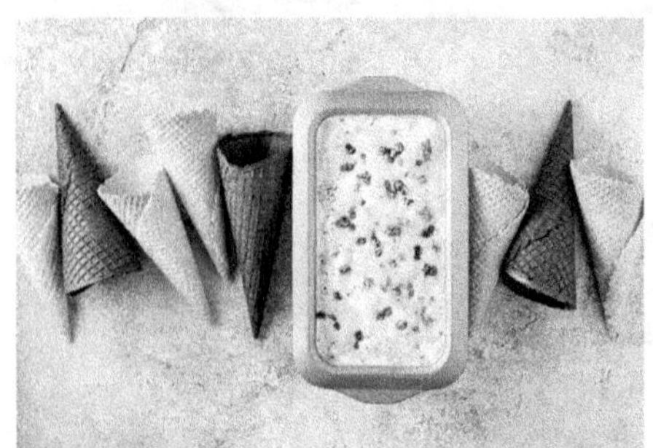

Preparation Time: 10 minutes
Cooking Time: 5 minutes
Serves: 6
Ingredients:

- ½ cup Greek yogurt
- 2 tbsp chocolate chips
- 2 tsp honey
- 3 tbsp creamy almond butter

Directions:

In a bowl, add yogurt, honey, and 2 tablespoons of almond butter and stir until completely mixed.

Spread the yogurt mixture evenly onto a parchment-lined baking sheet.

Sprinkle with chocolate chips and drizzle with remaining almond butter on top. Place in the freezer for 1 hour to completely freeze.

Break into pieces and serve.

Nutritional Data: 85 calories | 6.45g carbs | 5.29g fat | 3.95g protein | 40mg sodium

2-Baked Apples with Cinnamon

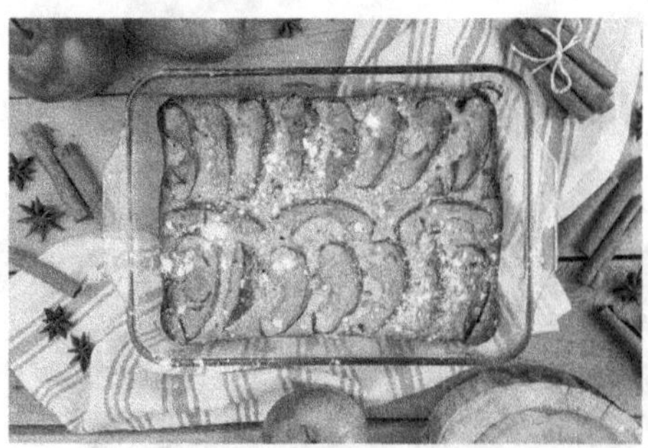

Preparation Time: 10 minutes
Cooking Time: 35 minutes
Serves: 4
Ingredients:

- 3 apples, cored & cut into ¼-inch thick slices
- 3 tbsp date sugar
- ½ tsp cinnamon
- 1 ½ tbsp lemon juice
- 1/3 cup maple syrup

Directions:

Preheat the oven to 350° F.

In a bowl, mix together maple syrup, lemon juice, and cinnamon. Add apple slices and mix until well coated.

Transfer apple slices to the baking dish and bake in preheated oven for 30 minutes.

Sprinkle date sugar over apple slices and bake for 5 minutes more. Remove from oven and allow to cool for 10 minutes.

Serve and enjoy.

Nutritional Data: 164 calories | 42.92g carbs | 0.27g fat | 0.4g protein | 5mg sodium

3-Dark Chocolate and Almond Clusters

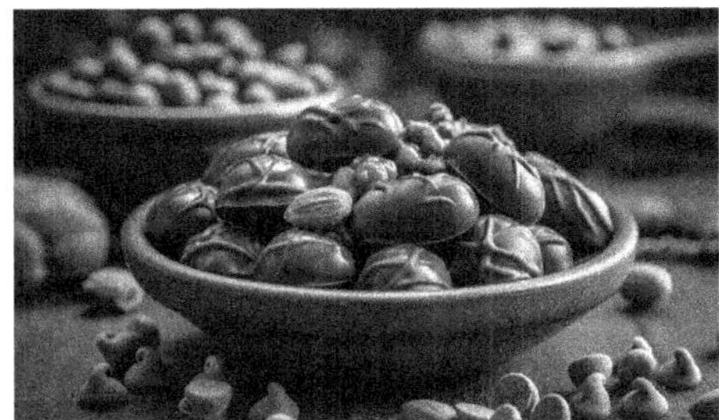

Preparation Time: 10 minutes
Cooking Time: 5 minutes
Serves: 24
Ingredients:

- 1 lb almonds, roasted
- 12 oz chocolate chips

Directions:

Line baking sheet with parchment paper and set aside.

Add chocolate chips into microwave-safe bowl and microwave for 30 seconds or until chocolate is melted. Remove from oven and stir until chocolate is smooth.

Add almonds to melted chocolate and stir until almonds are coated.

Using a spoon, scoop clusters of the almonds onto the baking sheet and allow to set completely.

Serve and enjoy.

Nutritional Data: 180 calories | 13.71g carbs | 12.71g fat | 4.73g protein | 59mg sodium

4-Berry and Yogurt Popsicles

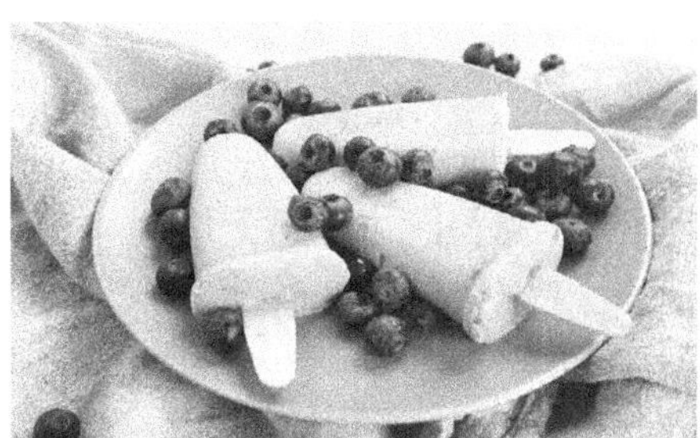

Preparation Time: 5 minutes
Cooking Time: 5 minutes
Serves: 10
Ingredients:

- 1 cup unsweetened coconut yogurt
- 1 cup raspberries
- ½ cup blackberries
- ½ cup blueberries
- 1 cup strawberries
- 2 tbsp maple syrup

Directions:

Add yogurt, berries, and maple syrup into blender and blend until smooth.

Pour the blended mixture into popsicle mold and place in the freezer overnight.

Serve and enjoy.

Nutritional Data: 66 calories | 16.44g carbs | 0.18g fat | 0.73g protein | 27mg sodium

5-Chia Seed Pudding

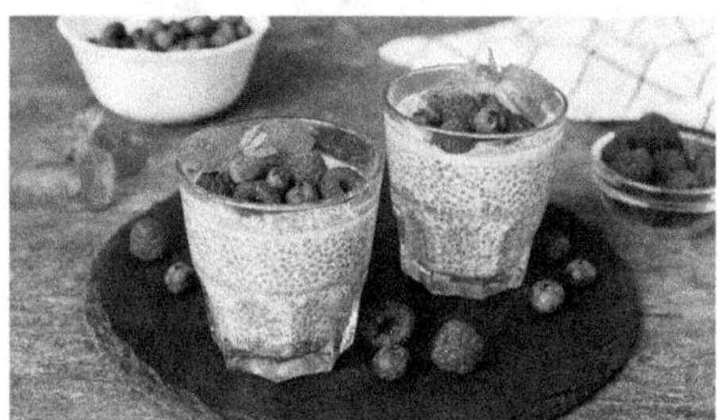

Preparation Time: 5 minutes
Cooking Time: 5 minutes
Serves: 4
Ingredients:

- ¼ cup chia seeds
- 1 tsp vanilla
- 2 tbsp maple syrup
- 1 cup Greek yogurt
- ¾ cup unsweetened almond milk
- 2 tbsp almonds, toasted & sliced
- ¼ cup blueberries
- ¼ cup raspberries
- ¼ cup strawberries, sliced

Directions:

In a bowl, mix together almond milk, yogurt, maple syrup, and vanilla. Add chia seeds and stir well. Cover and place in refrigerator overnight.

Spoon pudding into four serving glasses and top with almonds and berries.

Serve and enjoy.

Nutritional Data: 192 calories | 27.78g carbs | 6.48g fat | 7.17g protein | 50mg sodium

6-Banana Ice Cream

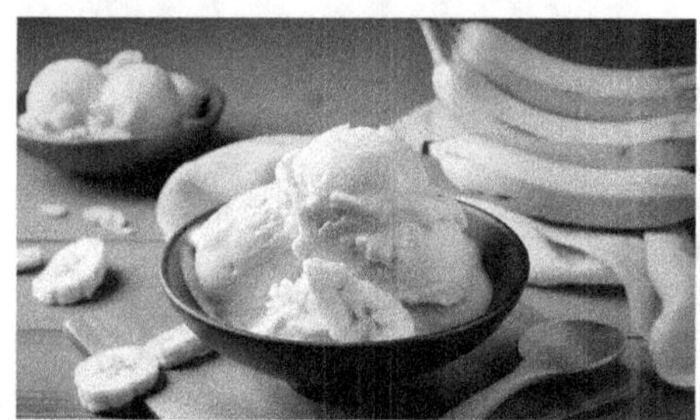

Preparation Time: 10 minutes
Cooking Time: 5 minutes
Serves: 2
Ingredients:

- 2 frozen bananas, cut into pieces
- 2 tsp maple syrup
- 2 tbsp unsweetened almond milk

Directions:

Add bananas, maple syrup, and almond milk into food processor and process until thick and creamy.

Serve immediately and enjoy.

Nutritional Data: 113 calories | 26.53g carbs | 0.96g fat | 3.12g protein | 14mg sodium

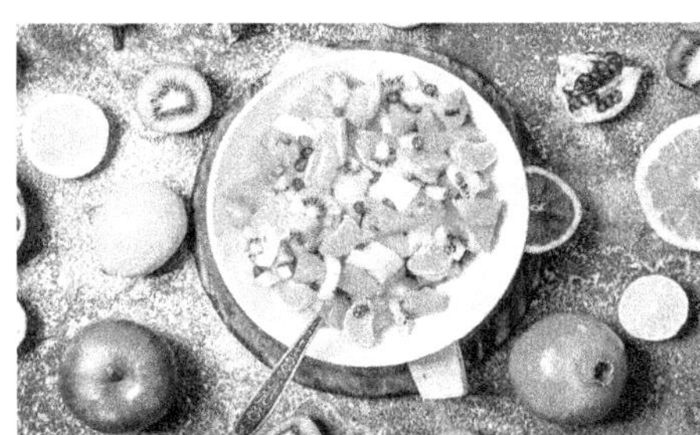

Preparation Time: 10 minutes
Cooking Time: 5 minutes
Serves: 8
Ingredients:

- 2 cups bananas, sliced
- ½ cup blueberries
- ½ cup raspberries
- 1 cup grapes, sliced
- ½ cup pomegranate arils
- 2 cups oranges
- 2 kiwis, peeled & sliced
- 1 pineapple, peeled & chopped
- For dressing:
- 1 tbsp poppy seeds
- 3 tbsp honey
- 3 tbsp fresh lemon juice

Directions:

Add all fruits into mixing bowl and mix well.

In a small bowl, whisk together lemon juice, honey, and poppy seeds and pour over the fruits.

Toss well and serve.

Nutritional Data: 253 calories | 63.15g carbs | 1.4g fat | 2.79g protein | 6mg sodium

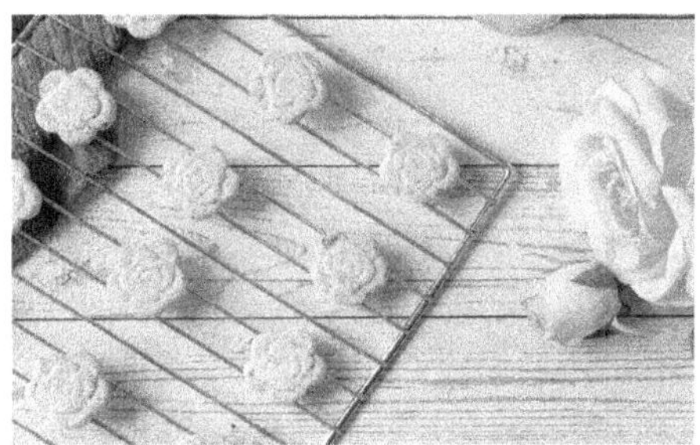

Preparation Time: 10 minutes
Cooking Time: 15 minutes
Serves: 15
Ingredients:

- 3 eggs whites
- 1 ½ cups unsweetened shredded coconut
- 1 tsp vanilla
- 1 tbsp coconut flour
- ½ cup erythritol

Directions:

Preheat the oven to 375° F.

Line baking sheet with parchment paper and set aside.

In a mixing bowl, beat the egg whites until foamy then add erythritol and beat on high speed until stiff peaks form.

Add vanilla and coconut flour and mix until just combined.

Add shredded coconut and fold gently.

Drop the batter by heaping tablespoons onto the prepared baking sheet and bake in preheated oven for 15 minutes. Remove from oven and allow to cool for 5 minutes.

Serve and enjoy.

Nutritional Data: 9 calories | 1.01g carbs | 0.06g fat | 0.9g protein | 37mg sodium

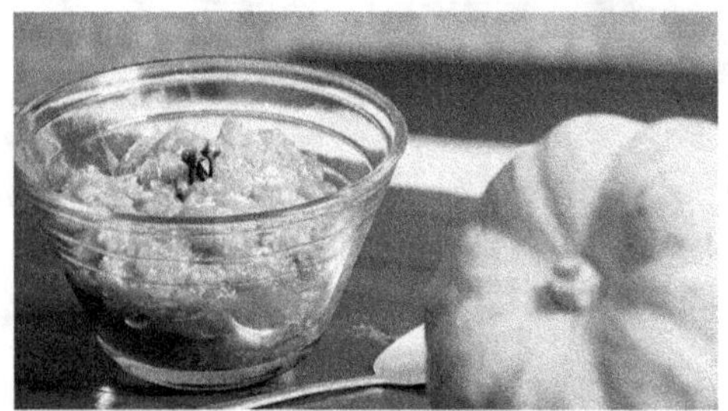

Preparation Time: 10 minutes
Cooking Time: 25 minutes
Serves: 6
Ingredients:

- 2 eggs
- 1 cup pumpkin puree
- 2 cups rolled oats
- 1 tsp cinnamon
- 2 tsp pumpkin pie spice
- 1 tsp vanilla
- ¼ cup maple syrup
- ¼ cup coconut oil, melted
- ¾ cup unsweetened almond milk
- ½ cup pecans, toasted & chopped

Directions:

Preheat the oven to 350° F.

Lightly grease 8-inch baking dish with cooking spray and set aside.

In a mixing bowl, mix together eggs, vanilla, maple syrup, coconut oil, almond milk, and pumpkin puree until smooth.

Add oats, cinnamon, pumpkin pie spice, and pecans and stir until well combined.

Add oatmeal mixture to the prepared baking dish and bake in preheated oven for 20–25 minutes.

Serve and enjoy.

Nutritional Data: 423 calories | 37.57g carbs | 30.54g fat | 15.28g protein | 109mg sodium

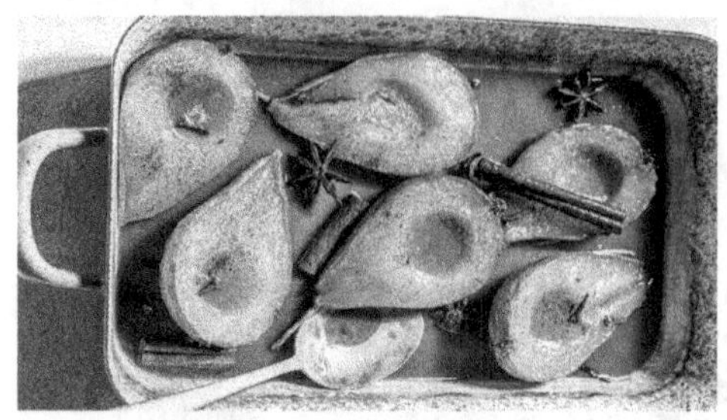

Preparation Time: 10 minutes
Cooking Time: 25 minutes
Serves: 8
Ingredients:

- 4 pears, sliced
- 2 tbsp honey
- 2 tsp cinnamon

Directions:

Preheat the oven to 375° F.

Arrange the pears in the baking dish and sprinkle cinnamon on top of the pears.

Bake in preheated oven for 25 minutes.

Drizzle with honey and serve.

Nutritional Data: 54 calories | 14.17g carbs | 0.21g fat | 0.48g protein | 0mg sodium

11-Greek Yogurt with Honey and Nuts

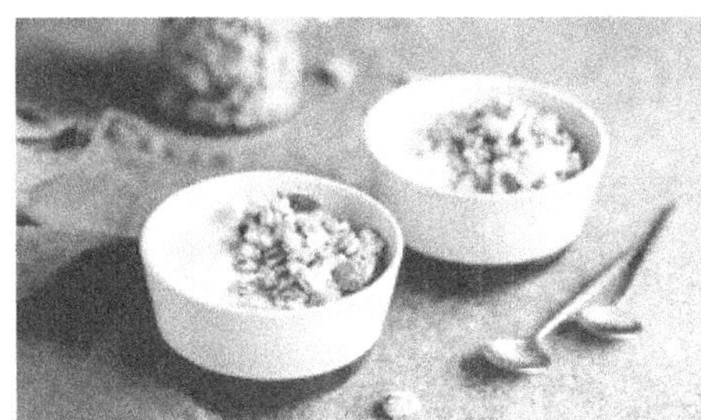

Preparation Time: 5 minutes
Cooking Time: 5 minutes
Serves: 2
Ingredients:

- 2 cups Greek yogurt
- 1 tbsp walnuts, toasted & chopped
- 1 tbsp almonds, toasted & chopped
- 4 tbsp honey

Directions:

Divide yogurt into two serving bowls.

Drizzle with honey and top with chopped nuts.

Serve and enjoy.

Nutritional Data: 288 calories | 43.21g carbs | 3.49g fat | 24.12g protein | 83mg sodium

12-Chocolate-Covered Strawberries

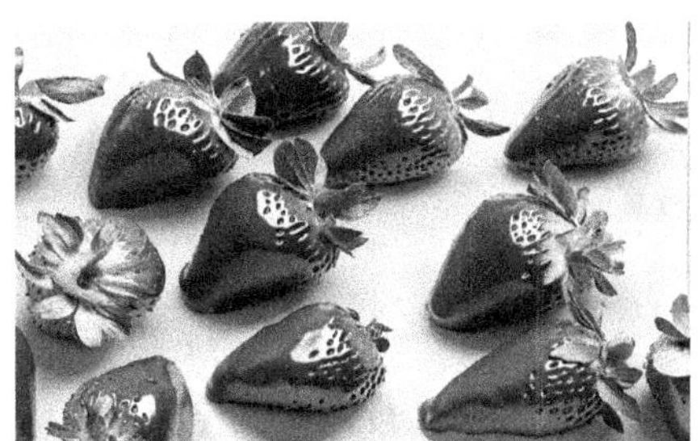

Preparation Time: 5 minutes
Cooking Time: 5 minutes
Serves: 8
Ingredients:

- 1 lb fresh strawberries, washed & patted dry with paper towels
- 2 tbsp butter
- 6 oz unsweetened chocolate chips

Directions:

Line cookie sheet with parchment paper and set aside.

Add chocolate chips and butter in a microwave-safe bowl and microwave for 30 seconds or until the chocolate melts.

Remove from microwave and mix well.

Dip each strawberry in melted chocolate to cover and place onto a prepared cookie sheet.

Place coated strawberries in the fridge for 2 hours.

Serve and enjoy

Nutritional Data: 149 calories | 18.82g carbs | 7.96g fat | 1.52g protein | 112mg sodium

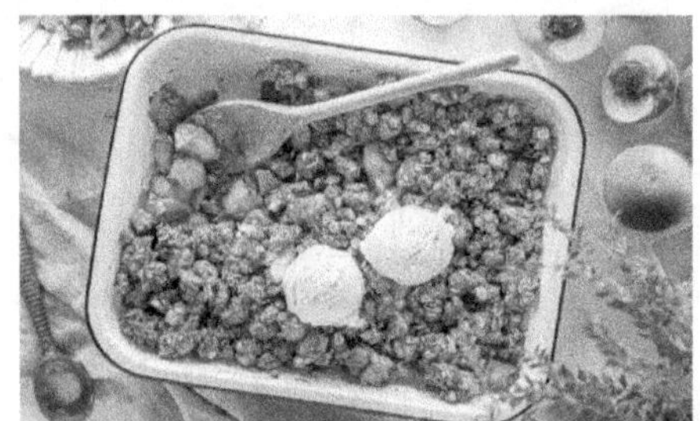

Preparation Time: 10 minutes
Cooking Time: 35 minutes
Serves: 6
Ingredients:

- 1 ¼ cups rolled oats
- 1 ½ lbs ripe peaches, sliced
- 1 tsp cinnamon
- 4 tbsp maple syrup
- 4 tbsp coconut oil, melted
- ½ cup almond flour

Directions:

Preheat the oven to 350° F.

Arrange peach slices into the baking dish.

Mix together oats, cinnamon, maple syrup, oil, and almond flour and spread evenly over the peaches.

Bake the peach crisp in preheated oven for 35 minutes.

Serve and enjoy.

Nutritional Data: 247 calories | 44.89g carbs | 10.62g fat | 3.94g protein | 9mg sodium

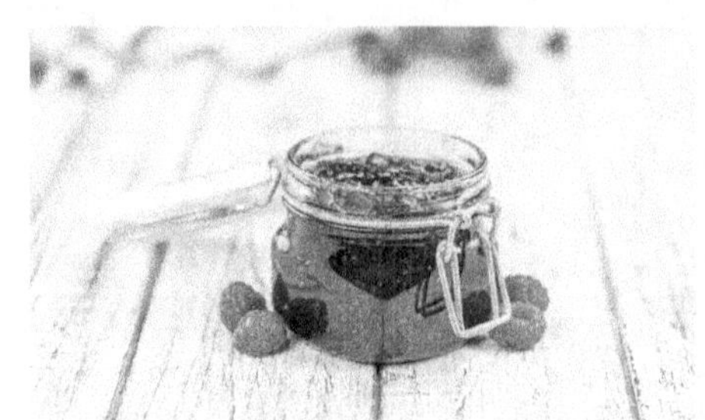

Preparation Time: 10 minutes
Cooking Time: 10 minutes
Serves: 12
Ingredients:

- 1 cup raspberries
- 1 ½ tbsp maple syrup
- 1 tsp chia seeds

Directions:

Add raspberries into a saucepan and cook over medium-high heat for 5 minutes or until softened. Gently mash raspberries using a spoon.

Add maple syrup and chia seeds and let the jam simmer for 10 minutes or until thickened. Remove from heat.

Let it cool completely then store in an airtight container in the fridge for up to 2 weeks.

Nutritional Data: 28 calories | 6.8g carbs | 0.13g fat | 0.23g protein | 1mg sodium

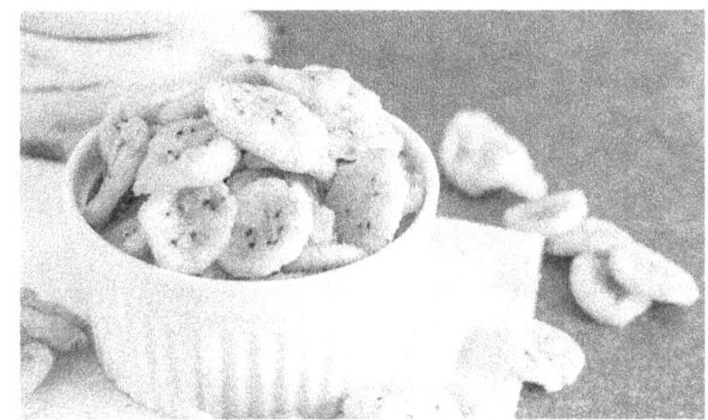

Preparation Time: 5 minutes
Cooking Time: 2 hours
Serves: 40 chips
Ingredients:

- 2 bananas, cut into 1/8-inch-thick coins
- ¼ cup water
- 1 tbsp fresh lemon juice

Directions:

Preheat the oven to 250° F.

Line baking sheet with parchment paper and set aside.

In a small bowl, mix water and lemon juice.

Arrange banana slices onto baking sheet and brush with water-lemon mixture.

Bake in preheated oven for 2 hours. Flip halfway through. Remove from oven and allow to cool completely.

Serve and enjoy.

Nutritional Data: 8 calories | 2g carbs | 0.01g fat | 0.05g protein | 0mg sodium

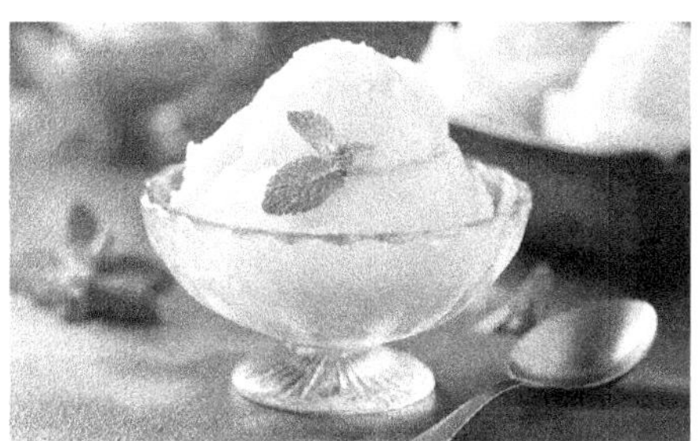

Preparation Time: 10 minutes
Cooking Time: 5 minutes
Serves: 2
Ingredients:

- 4 cups frozen pineapple
- 1 ½ tbsp honey

Directions:

Add frozen pineapple and honey in a blender and blend until smooth and creamy.

Serve immediately and enjoy.

Nutritional Data: 469 calories | 121.76g carbs | 0.49g fat | 2.01g protein | 10mg sodium

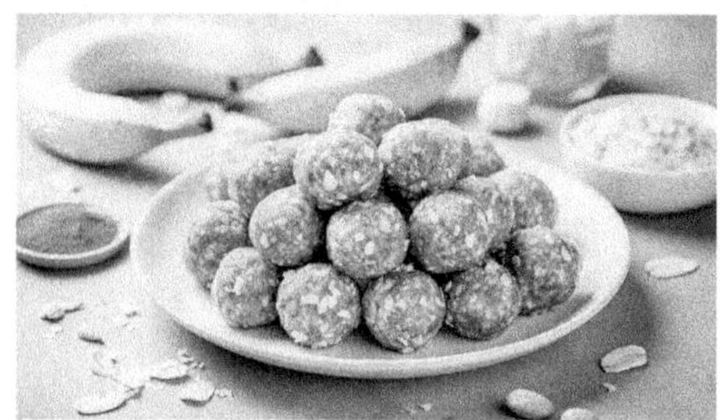

Preparation Time: 10 minutes
Cooking Time: 10 minutes
Serves: 25 banana bites
Ingredients:

- 3 bananas, cut into slices
- 2 tbsp maple syrup
- 2 tbsp coconut oil
- 1/3 cup unsweetened almond butter

Directions:

In a small pot, add almond butter, maple syrup, and coconut oil and heat over medium heat just until coconut oil is melted. Remove from heat and whisk well to combine.

Dip each banana slice in almond butter mixture and coat well.

Place coated banana slices onto a parchment-lined baking sheet and place in the freezer for 2 hours.

Serve and enjoy.

Nutritional Data: 75 calories | 12.29g carbs | 3.14g fat | 1.16g protein | 8mg sodium

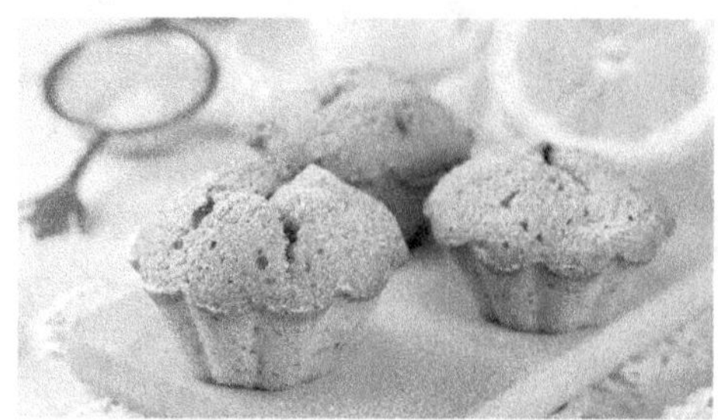

Preparation Time: 10 minutes
Cooking Time: 25 minutes
Serves: 9
Ingredients:

- 3 eggs
- 1 tsp lemon zest
- ¼ cup lemon juice
- 1 tbsp poppy seeds
- 1 tsp vanilla
- ½ cup canola oil
- 2 tsp baking powder
- ½ cup erythritol
- 2 ¾ cups almond flour

Directions:

Preheat the oven to 350° F.

Lightly grease muffin pan with cooking spray and set aside.

In a mixing bowl, whisk eggs with lemon zest, canola oil, and vanilla.

Add almond flour, lemon juice, baking powder, and erythritol and mix until just combined.

Add poppy seeds and fold well.

Spoon batter into the prepared muffin pan and bake in preheated oven for 25 minutes. Remove from oven and let them cool completely.

Serve and enjoy.

Nutritional Data: 169 calories | 1.78g carbs | 15.94g fat | 3.27g protein | 35mg sodium

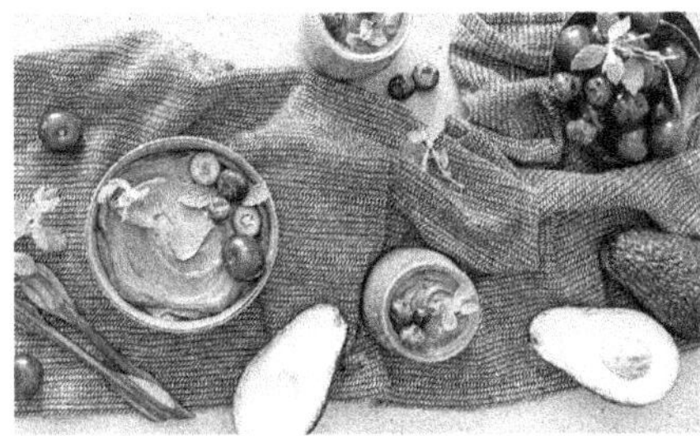

Preparation Time: 5 minutes
Cooking Time: 5 minutes
Serves: 4
Ingredients:

- 1 large avocado, flesh scooped out
- 6 ½ tbsp maple syrup
- ½ cup unsweetened almond milk
- ½ cup cashew nuts
- ¼ cup unsweetened cocoa powder

Directions:

Add avocado flesh and remaining ingredients into blender and blend until smooth.

Spoon the mousse into serving glasses and place in the refrigerator for 30 minutes.

Serve and enjoy.

Nutritional Data: 285 calories | 36.89g carbs | 16.17g fat | 4.9g protein | 79mg sodium

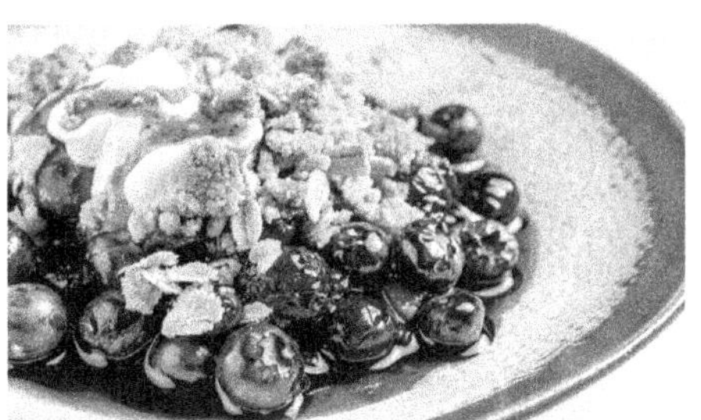

Preparation Time: 10 minutes
Cooking Time: 45 minutes
Serves: 6
Ingredients:

- 5 cups frozen berries
- 2 tsp cinnamon
- 3 tbsp water
- 3 tbsp maple syrup
- For crumble:
- ½ cup almond flour
- 1 cup oats
- ¼ cup maple syrup
- ¼ cup coconut oil, melted
- ¼ cup walnuts, chopped
- ¼ cup almonds, chopped

Directions:

Preheat the oven to 350° F.

In a mixing bowl, toss berries with cinnamon, water, and maple syrup.

Transfer berries into 8x8-inch greased baking dish.

For crumble: In a separate bowl, mix oats, maple syrup, coconut oil, cinnamon, almonds, walnuts, and almond flour and spread over berries.

Bake in preheated oven for 45 minutes or until lightly golden brown.

Serve and enjoy.

Nutritional Data: 386 calories | 58.39g carbs | 17.68g fat | 7.64g protein | 95mg sodium

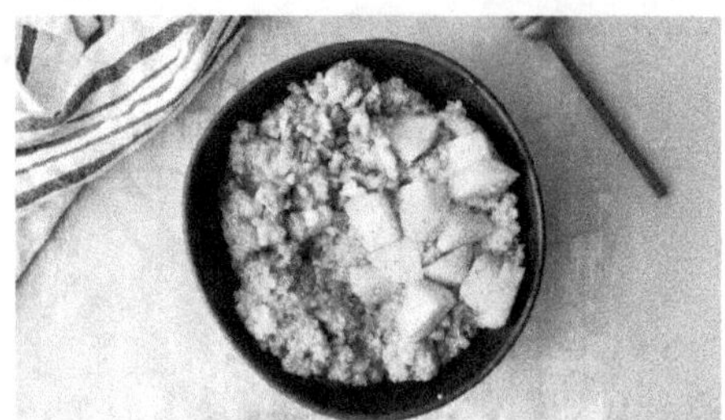

Preparation Time: 10 minutes
Cooking Time: 25 minutes
Serves: 2
Ingredients:

- ½ cup quinoa, rinsed & drained
- 2 tsp cinnamon
- 2 apples, cored & chopped
- 1 ½ cups water
- 2 tbsp honey

Directions:

Add quinoa, apples, and water to a saucepan and bring to a boil, cover and simmer over low heat for 20–25 minutes.

Add cinnamon and stir well.

Transfer quinoa into two serving bowls and drizzle with honey.

Serve and enjoy.

Nutritional Data: 321 calories | 71.8g carbs | 2.92g fat | 6.64g protein | 9mg sodium

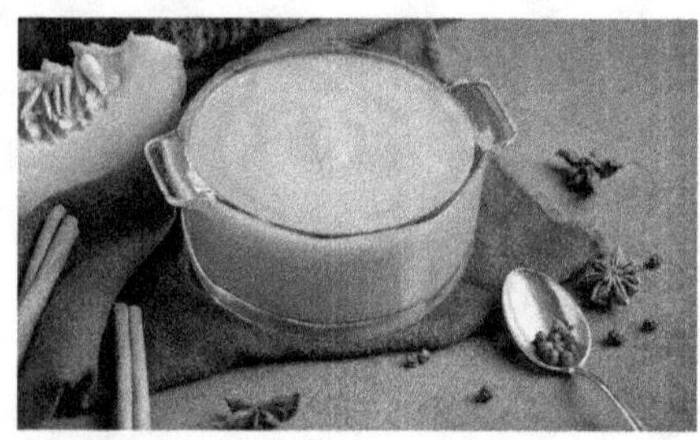

Preparation Time: 5 minutes
Cooking Time: 5 minutes
Serves: 2
Ingredients:

- ½ cup pumpkin puree
- 1 tsp pumpkin pie spice
- 1 tsp vanilla
- 2 tbsp maple syrup
- 1 cup unsweetened almond milk
- ½ cup pumpkin puree
- ½ cup Greek yogurt
- 1 frozen banana
- 3–4 ice cubes

Directions:

Add pumpkin puree and remaining ingredients into blender and blend until smooth.

Serve and enjoy.

Nutritional Data: 653 calories | 79.6g carbs | 31.6g fat | 23.93g protein | 253mg sodium

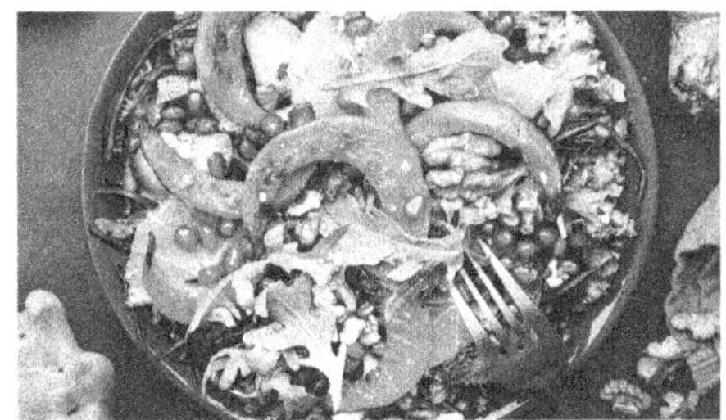

Preparation Time: 10 minutes
Cooking Time: 5 minutes
Serves: 4
Ingredients:
- 6 dates, pitted & sliced
- 4 oranges, peeled, pith removed, and cut into slices
- 1 tbsp honey
- ¼ cup orange juice
- 1 chili pepper, diced
- ¼ cup pomegranate seeds

Directions:

In a mixing bowl, mix dates, oranges, chili pepper, and pomegranate seeds.

Mix together honey and orange juice and drizzle over the salad.

Toss well and serve.

Nutritional Data: 195 calories | 47.21g carbs | 0.59g fat | 2.6g protein | 7mg sodium

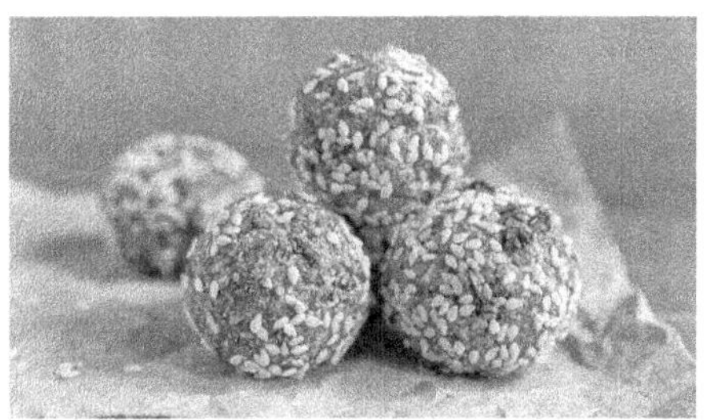

Preparation Time: 10 minutes
Cooking Time: 10 minutes
Serves: 15 energy balls
Ingredients:
- 1 cup walnuts
- 1 ½ cups dried figs, soaked in warm water for 10 minutes
- ½ tsp cinnamon
- 1 tsp maple syrup
- 1 tsp vanilla
- 3 tbsp hemp seeds

Directions:

Add walnuts to a food processor and process until coarsely chopped.

Add hemp seeds, cinnamon, maple syrup, and vanilla and process until combined.

Drain figs well and add to the food processor and process until sticky dough forms.

Make equal shapes of balls from the mixture and place onto a plate. Place in refrigerator for 20 minutes.

Serve and enjoy.

Nutritional Data: 84 calories | 11g carbs | 4.52g fat | 1.67g protein | 2mg sodium

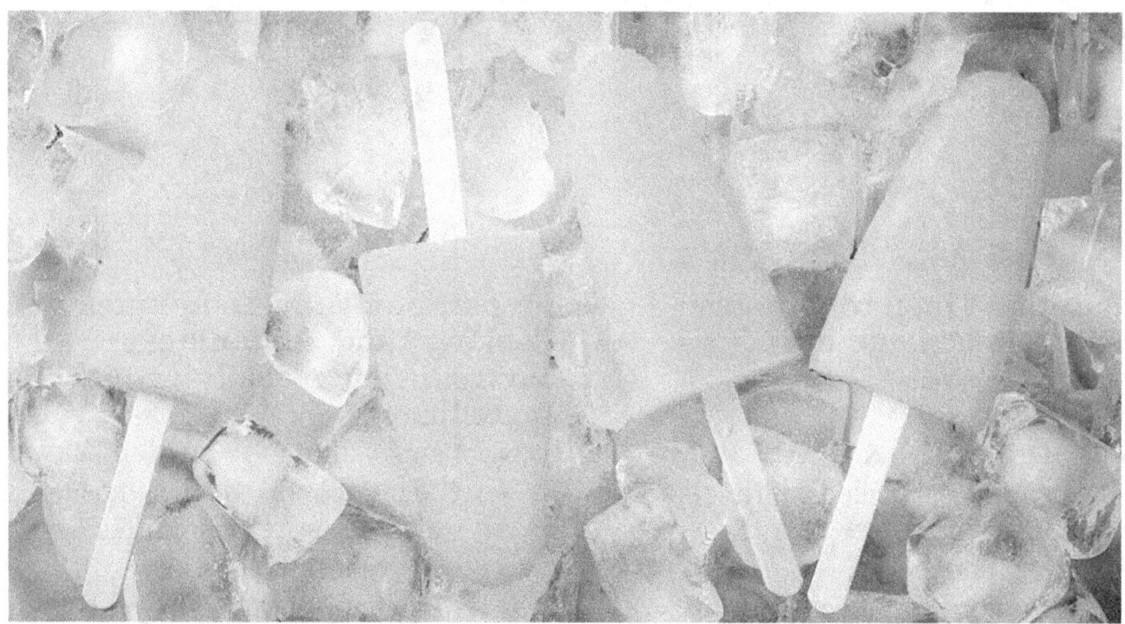

Preparation Time: 5 minutes
Cooking Time: 5 minutes
Serves: 6
Ingredients:

- 2 frozen bananas
- 1 tbsp cocoa powder
- 2 tbsp peanut butter
- 1 cup unsweetened soymilk

Directions:

Add frozen bananas and remaining ingredients into blender and blend until smooth.

Pour the blended mixture into popsicle mold and place in the freezer overnight.

Serve and enjoy.

Nutritional Data: 145 calories | 32.69g carbs | 1.99g fat | 2.8g protein | 101mg sodium

Plan and Prepare DASH Meals for 30 Days

1. **First, you need to understand the dietary guidelines:**
   Include more fruits, vegetables, and whole grains in your diet.
   Always favor low-fat or fat-free dairy products, poultry, fish, beans, nuts, and vegetable oils.
   Limit consumption of saturated fats, red meats, sweets, and unhealthy sugary drinks.
   Reduce daily sodium intake to less than 2,300 mg per day — 1,500 mg per day for even better results.

2. **Set your daily or weekly nutritional goal**
   Develop daily and weekly nutritional goals, marking foods and groups you should consume within the acceptable range. For example, you can aim for 4–5 servings of vegetables, 4–5 servings of fruits, and 6–8 servings of grains per day.

3. **Make a 30-day menu**
   Prior preparation of what you will eat at every meal will help you stick to your plan. The menu should have different recipes for breakfast, lunch, dinner, and snacks to keep you from repeating and losing interest. In addition, there are DASH diet recipes compiled by Eating Well that you can draw from for varied and customized mix-and-match options for meals.

4. **Make shopping lists in advance**
   Compile weekly shopping lists based on your menu. You will need to gather some fresh produce, whole grains, and low-fat dairy products. Organize your list by food categories (fruits, vegetables, proteins, etc.) to streamline the shopping process. It is helpful to check pantry staples such as oils, vinegar, spices, grains, and canned goods before each trip so that you can avoid purchasing more than you need. Batch grocery shopping and batch meals can save a lot of time.

5. **Meal preparation and batch cooking**
   Try to prepare multiple meals at once that can be refrigerated or frozen and then easily reheated. Meals such as soups, stews, or casseroles work best when planning to batch cook. Preparing and storing multiple meals can make meal execution throughout the week much easier and may be the extra motivation you need to comply with the DASH diet.

6. **Keep an eye on portion size**
   Correct portion sizes are important, especially when it comes to calorie consumption. In the DASH diet, portions tend to be larger for lower-calorie, bulkier foods. Use measuring cups and digital scales to measure out exact portion sizes to

ensure you stay within the recommended portions of each food group on the DASH eating plan.

7. Stay Hydrated

In addition to eating a nutrient-rich diet, hydration plays an important role when you are following the DASH diet. Most of us need 8 to 10 cups of water daily from foods and beverages to keep our bodies hydrated. Avoid high-calorie and sweetened drinks to limit your carb intake. Proper hydration supports your digestive process, regulates your metabolic process, and also helps in blood pressure regulation.

8. Be flexible and adapt it

Based on what you like or dislike and what you can or cannot find in the grocery stores due to the seasonal availability of certain ingredients, flexibility can help you enjoy this diet through its 30 days.

9. Keep a food diary

Keep a food diary to track your progress. This way, you can also document your adherence to the diet, how it worked for you, and generally how this dieting period affected and changed your life.

10. Engage Support Networks

Eat your DASH meals with others and allow them to share feedback with you about how your cooking could be improved or simply provide motivation for you to stick to the plan. You can even share the experience with someone else who would also like to give the DASH diet a try and perhaps experiment with your recipes together. Joining DASH diet communities or forums online can also be beneficial. These communities will offer you support and great recipe ideas.

The following are holistic tips to guide you through eating out on the DASH diet:

1. **Scan the menu carefully for dishes:** While enjoying an evening dining out, consider looking at the list of foods that are compliant with fresh fruits, vegetables, whole grains, lean proteins, and low-fat dairy.

2. **Pay attention to sodium:** Considering that the DASH diet emphasizes sodium reduction, you may ask the server to prepare your dish with low-sodium or sodium-free sauce. Avoid additional salt and ask if they can serve it with a salt-substitute sauce.

3. **Be wise in the drinks you pick:** Your best choices are water, herbal tea, and coffee. They are perfect for the DASH diet — less of the fatty dairy idea, and also for not drinking so many of your calories in the form of salty or sugary drinks.

4. **Choose nutrient-rich foods:** When you look at the menu, always choose nutrient-rich foods, such as fresh fish, other seafood, beef, chicken, fruits, and vegetables. This style of eating will help you achieve your DASH-diet goals in the long run and keep you healthy.

5. **Choose Beverages Wisely:** While eating out on the DASH diet, avoid sugary sodas, energy drinks, fruit juices with added sugars, alcoholic beverages, and high-calorie coffee drinks with syrups and whipped cream. Some of these drinks are high in calories, sugars, and bad fats, which do not align with DASH diet goals.

6. **Don't forget to customize your order:** Make a no-added-salt request and utilize other seasonings, which can include light soy sauce. Also, communicate your dietary preferences to the server to ensure the meal fits within the stipulations of your DASH diet.

7. **Highlight Fresh Produce and Grill:** While eating out, choose products based on fresh, non-processed ingredients and pick grilled or steamed dishes rather than deep-fried or served with sauce. That is consistent with the DASH diet's focus on whole meals and easier means of preparation.

Day 1
- Breakfast: Blueberry Oatmeal
- Lunch: Mediterranean Chickpea Salad
- Dinner: Baked Salmon with Lemon and Herbs

Day 2
- Breakfast: Avocado Toast
- Lunch: Quinoa and Black Bean-Stuffed Bell Peppers
- Dinner: Quinoa-Stuffed Bell Peppers

Day 3
- Breakfast: Greek Yogurt Parfait
- Lunch: Grilled Chicken Caesar Salad
- Dinner: Grilled Chicken with Roasted Vegetables

Day 4
- Breakfast: Veggie Omelet
- Lunch: Turkey and Avocado Wrap
- Dinner: Turkey Chili

Day 5
- Breakfast: Whole Grain Pancakes
- Lunch: Vegetable Stir-Fry with Brown Rice
- Dinner: Lemon Garlic Shrimp with Brown Rice

Day 6
- Breakfast: Chia Seed Pudding
- Lunch: Salmon and Quinoa Salad
- Dinner: Vegetable Stir-Fry with Tofu

Day 7
- Breakfast: Banana Smoothie
- Lunch: Whole Wheat Pasta Primavera
- Dinner: Eggplant Parmesan

Day 8
- Breakfast: Egg and Spinach Breakfast Wrap
- Lunch: Greek Yogurt Chicken Salad
- Dinner: Pesto Zucchini Noodles with Cherry Tomatoes

Day 9

Day 10
- Breakfast: Apple Cinnamon-Baked Oatmeal
- Lunch: Veggie and Hummus Wrap
- Dinner: Baked Chicken Parmesan

Day 11
- Breakfast: Ricotta & Berry Toast
- Lunch: Tuna and White Bean Salad
- Dinner: Salmon with Roasted Asparagus

Day 12
- Breakfast: Sweet Potato Hash
- Lunch: Black Bean and Corn Quesadillas
- Dinner: Vegetable and Lentil Shepherd's Pie

Day 13
- Breakfast: Mediterranean Breakfast Bowl
- Lunch: Stuffed Zucchini Boats
- Dinner: Mushroom and Spinach Risotto

Day 14
- Breakfast: Spinach and Mushroom Frittata
- Lunch: Vegetable and Lentil Curry
- Dinner: Baked Cod with Mediterranean Salsa

Day 15
- Breakfast: Peanut Butter Banana Smoothie
- Lunch: Mushroom and Spinach Quesadillas
- Dinner: Stuffed Acorn Squash

Day 16
- Breakfast: Oatmeal Banana Muffins
- Lunch: Caprese Quinoa Salad
- Dinner: Turkey Meatballs with Marinara Sauce

Day 17
- Breakfast: Egg & Veggie Breakfast Burrito
- Lunch: Turkey and Vegetable Lettuce

- Breakfast: Quinoa Breakfast Bowl
- Lunch: Lentil Soup
- Dinner: Lentil and Vegetable Curry

Day 18

- Breakfast: Cottage Cheese with Fruit
- Lunch: Egg Salad Lettuce Wraps
- Dinner: Black Bean and Sweet Potato Tacos

Day 19

- Breakfast: Pumpkin Spice Overnight Oats
- Lunch: Veggie and Brown Rice Sushi Rolls
- Dinner: Spinach and Mushroom-Stuffed Chicken Breast

Day 20

- Breakfast: Turkey Sausage Breakfast Sandwich
- Lunch: Sweet Potato and Black Bean Salad
- Dinner: Eggplant and Zucchini Lasagna

Day 21

- Breakfast: Yogurt and Berry Smoothie Bowl
- Lunch: Chicken and Vegetable Skewers
- Dinner: Pork Tenderloin with Apple Cider Glaze

Day 22

- Breakfast: Egg and Cheese Breakfast Quesadilla
- Lunch: Quinoa and Kale Salad
- Dinner: Vegetable and Tofu Stir-Fry

Day 23

- Breakfast: Almond Butter and Banana Toast
- Lunch: Black Bean and Vegetable Burrito Bowl
- Dinner: Salmon with Mango Salsa

Wraps
- Dinner: Lemon Herb Chicken Skewers

Day 24

- Breakfast: Berry Quinoa Breakfast Bowl
- Lunch: Mediterranean Veggie Wrap
- Dinner: Mushroom and Spinach Quinoa

Day 25

- Breakfast: Cranberry Orange Muffins
- Lunch: Avocado Corn Tomato Salad
- Dinner: Turkey and Vegetable Skillet

Day 26

- Breakfast: Blueberry Oatmeal
- Lunch: Mediterranean Chickpea Salad
- Dinner: Baked Salmon with Lemon and Herbs

Day 27

- Breakfast: Avocado Toast
- Lunch: Quinoa and Black Bean-Stuffed Bell Peppers
- Dinner: Quinoa-Stuffed Bell Peppers

Day 28

- Breakfast: Greek Yogurt Parfait
- Lunch: Grilled Chicken Caesar Salad
- Dinner: Grilled Chicken with Roasted Vegetables

Day 29

- Breakfast: Veggie Omelet
- Lunch: Turkey and Avocado Wrap
- Dinner: Turkey Chili

Day 30

- Breakfast: Whole Grain Pancakes
- Lunch: Vegetable Stir-Fry with Brown Rice
- Dinner: Lemon Garlic Shrimp with Brown Rice

Conclusion

The DASH (Dietary Approaches to Stop Hypertension) diet is one of the most well-researched diets that has a large and long list of studies that support and validate it very well. Numerous clinical trials, meta-analyses, and systematic reviews that are both long-term and well-controlled have provided consistent, overwhelmingly positive results regarding the cardiovascular benefits of the DASH diet, and it is now considered to be the best non-pharmacological nutrition therapy for blood pressure reduction and heart failure treatment. This kind of diet is in line with the quality and quantity of foods recommended for a healthy diet and also the type of diet that is best for the management of high blood pressure.

The DASH Diet works best with high blood pressure. It seems to be very clear that the DASH Diet reduces blood pressure the most effectively in people who have high blood pressure. However, the good news is that it seems that the effect is quite robust, and it certainly reduces blood pressure across several different subpopulations. I believe that many people could easily benefit from starting to eat a little bit more like the DASH Diet as just a small part of a comprehensive strategy to manage blood pressure. Another tenet of the DASH diet is that it stresses whole foods: a lot of fruits, vegetables, whole grains, lean proteins, and low-fat dairy. These types of food and nutrient patterns are well supported by most dietary guidelines for cardiovascular disease. So, it returns to the basics of how we should be eating to prevent heart disease, stroke, and other forms of cardiovascular disease. The last thing that I think is important is that the DASH diet improves other types of biomarkers of cardiovascular disease. Over the last several decades, a lot of the talk and science in nutrition has very much transformed to try to move away from dietary cholesterol and blood cholesterol being the primary culprits in cardiovascular disease to other types of biomarkers such as inflammation, oxidative stress, and vascular reactivity, and many other lipoprotein classes that I personally did not even know existed in the late 80s and the early 90s.

Many studies have shown an improvement in a number of these biomarkers with the DASH diet. In many cases, the final common pathway of heart disease starts with vascular injury or biomarkers of cardiovascular disease that serve as the canaries of early signs of future health issues. So, the DASH diet may be helpful not just in managing cardiovascular disease for people who already have heart disease, high blood pressure, or similarly, but very likely in preventing cardiovascular diseases in the first place. And that would make it a really powerful tool in the arsenal for nutrition in the cardiovascular world.

The positive benefits of the DASH diet are not limited to reduced blood pressure but also extends to other cardiovascular risk factors. Thus, people with hypertension can also experience diminished waist circumference and triglyceride concentration due to the DASH diet. Such an indication proves that the influence of the diet covers various cardiovascular health parameters and may be connected with a lesser chance of developing gout. It means that the DASH-diet approach is not just a strategy to deal with hypertension but a multi-beneficial tactic to solve several health-related problems.

The body of research supporting the DASH diet has persistently shown that this diet is universally beneficial for promoting health, particularly for controlling blood pressure. The DASH diet has also been acknowledged as an efficacious dietary pattern that may be useful as non-drug therapy in the management of heart failure. It has even been hinted that it is an inherently versatile diet that can be applied in practice for issues of cardiac health across the spectrum of patient populations and clinical scenarios.

To conclude, the DASH diet is a total dietary pattern that aligns with the recommended suggestions for blood pressure control and cardiovascular health promotion. It has been shown to produce good results such as a decrease in blood pressure BP, enhanced cardiovascular disease biomarkers and so extensive cardiovascular health outcomes due to the focus on whole foods, low-sodium content, and nutrient-dense ingredients. Therefore, DASH is a fantastic dietary prescription for hypertension patients as well as people striving to maintain or enhance cardiovascular health given its prevalence and diversity of benefits.

Reference Page

9 Health benefits of the DASH diet. (2024, April 2). Rupa Health. https://www.rupahealth.com/post/9-health-benefits-of-the-dash-diet

Brazier, Y. (2024, March 25). *The DASH diet: How does it work?*https://www.medicalnewstoday.com/articles/254836

DASH diet and high blood pressure. (2024, April 4). WebMD. https://www.webmd.com/hypertension-high-blood-pressure/dash-diet

DASH diet: Healthy eating to lower your blood pressure. (2023, May 25). Mayo Clinic. https://www.mayoclinic.org/healthy-lifestyle/nutrition-and-healthy-eating/in-depth/dash-diet/art-20048456

DASH diet: Tips for dining out. (2023, April 22). Middlesex Health. https://middlesexhealth.org/learning-center/articles/dash-diet-tips-for-dining-out#:~:text=Opt%20for%20healthier%20fare%2C%20such,such%20as%20cheese%20and%20dressing.

Mph, E. O. N. (2022, March 24). *DASH diet: Lower blood pressure, foods to avoid & Foods to eat.* MedicineNet. https://www.medicinenet.com/the_dash_diet/article.htm

Rd, H. W. (2018, October 17). *The complete beginner's guide to the DASH diet.* Healthline. https://www.healthline.com/nutrition/dash-diet#salt-restriction

Rust, R., Kleckner, C., & Samaan, S. (2021, March 19). *Dining Out on the DASH Diet dummies.* Dummies. https://www.dummies.com/article/body-mind-spirit/physical-health-well-being/diet-nutrition/dash-diet/dining-out-on-the-dash-diet-275619/

The DASH diet can help with high-blood pressure. (n.d.). Eufic. https://www.eufic.org/en/healthy-living/article/the-dash-diet-can-help-with-high-blood-pressure

Tips to tackling the DASH diet. (2024, March 27). National Kidney Foundation. https://www.kidney.org/atoz/content/Dash_Diet_Tips

Understanding the DASH diet: MedlinePlus Medical Encyclopedia. (n.d.). https://medlineplus.gov/ency/patientinstructions/000784.htm